About The Author

At the age of twenty-five, Leanne Chilton had a grand mal seizure in her sleep. She was told that she had epilepsy and would have to be on medication for the rest of her life. She was young, healthy, and quite active. She was in a good relationship with someone she loved very much, and was dreaming of success and a partner to share it with. She also believed that hard work and a positive attitude would keep her safe from life's misfortunes.

Bad things do happen to all of us, and it's not what you are or who you know that makes you a better person. It's how you deal with the tragedies that come into your life and what you make out of life's disappointments that enables you to move on.

Leanne was prompted to write *Seizure Free* while taking a vacation from school. It occurred to her that there were no books in the retail stores or in the libraries on how to survive brain surgery and epilepsy. Brain surgery was still relatively new, and patients and their families had only a few places to go for answers. Leanne wanted a book that would offer more to the world and that would break down the barriers between the "disabled" and the "non-disabled."

Today Leanne is thirty-six years old and four and a half years seizure free. She had brain surgery in April of '95 and completely came off medication by November of that year. She has written and published two books and started her own business. She is currently working on leading a balanced life.

This compelling account of courage and hope is as good as medicine. <u>Seizure Free</u> is an inspiring and very personal story of a young Texas woman who endured epilepsy--and prevailed. "My only hope was to put every bit of energy into being positive." Chilton went through several personal hells, for sure. And she speaks to the reader about them like a sister. In the end, we learn intimate and informative details about how to get through seizures and brain surgery. And get on with your life. Chilton had her first grand mal seizure at age 25. A few years later, she was seizure free, off medication and on her way with a new career. She tells what likely caused her problem, she shares the humiliation, and she takes readers through the life of a victim. The impact on loved ones, the secrets to keep, learning to trust doctors, the importance of a support system, medications and their effects. (Chilton includes web sites for some great Internet help). Readers learn details about MRI, CAT, PETT, EEG, and other modern diagnostics tools. "Your doctors may not be able to detect any abnormal brain wave activity. That doesn't mean that you're crazy, yet!" This isn't all warm and fuzzy. She had post-op depression, she felt fragile. The confusion of healing "made me sad and mad all over again." Then readers feel the forging of a new person, a new future. This book shares life on every page.

---The Book Reader

This book is dedicated with love to
Derek A. Bruce, M.D., my neurosurgeon
and friend, without whom, I wouldn't have
had a success story to tell or a reason to tell it.
Your strength, sensitivity, and humbleness
have been an inspiration to me that
no one can ever replace.
Thank You for giving me my life back!

Acknowledgments

I would like to thank my sister, Kay, for believing in me and for believing in my goals. You have a way of looking at life that can be very refreshing and rewarding when someone else's life is not going as planned. Thanks for seeing my strengths, thanks for always supporting my endeavors, and thanks for your contribution to this book!

I would like to thank my neurosurgeon, Derek A. Bruce, M.D., my epileptologist, Robert F. Leroy, M.D., my therapist, Kathie Beckman Smallwood, Ph.D., and my college advisor, Sinah Goode, Ph.D. Thank you for being in my life and for giving me something to believe in! I would like to add a special thanks to Derek Bruce for taking the time to write the foreword to my book. You have dedicated your life to your patients and to being the best neurosurgeon in the world! An inspiration and mentor in the medical field, and a positive role model for many!

I would also like to thank some people who were in my life at various times when I was having seizures and rehabilitating from surgery. These people include my parents, John P. and Shirley Chilton, my confidantes, Corky Enslin, Wendy, Donna A., Marilyn, Debra T., Debra B., Sandy, Donna H., Jean, Paige, my research nurse, Cynthia Felts, my aunt, Lelah, my brother and sister-in-law, Johnny and Alexandra, and my nephews and niece, JP, Levi, and Lauren.

FOREWORD

Seizure Free is one of these special books that will be helpful not only to those with epilepsy, their families, friends, and the physicians who share in their care, but also to the reading public. As a personal view of the journey through the onset of epilepsy, to the treatment, and finally to the cure of epileptic seizures, this book allows the reader to share in the ups and downs of that experience and to gain insight into the pain and pleasure of a real life drama. Leanne shares her experience in a way that is understandable and includes the reader as a companion on her journey.

Seizure Free should be required reading for all medical personnel involved in the care and treatment of people with epilepsy. As a neurosurgeon, I've learned an important lesson. The events most frightening and concerning for the patients are not always those that I would have expected. Leanne was recently in my office talking to a teenager who was scheduled for surgery the next day. The teenager and I had discussed all the dangers of surgery, yet it transpired when she was talking to Leanne that her real concern involved the pin head rest.* She was afraid the pin head rest would leave a big hole on her forehead. This would never have been broached with me. Leanne even confessed later that her fear was the arterial line that is inserted into the wrist and used to check blood pressure during surgery.

As a neurosurgeon my focus and concern is with the brain, but as a physician, my concern is with easing my patients' fears. This is a special book by a special person and will be of great value to all who read it regardless of their involvement with epilepsy. It is an insight into the strength and vibrancy of the human spirit!

Derek A. Bruce, M.D.
Pediatric Neurosurgery

---

*The pin head rest is used to hold the head in a stationary position during surgery. The skull is placed in the head rest and held secure by three pins that slightly penetrate the skull. The marks left on the skin from the pins are undetectable within a few weeks after surgery.

Contents

Introduction

I just feel like every pill I put into my body destroys me a little each day! And I block it out until I convince myself I feel good and just about that time, the seizures start again. I never know how long they'll last or how strong they'll be until they end. And then I'm sick again from all of the medication.

I'm writing this down because I don't ever want to look back and say it was easy; but I know that some day I will. And then I'll look at all I've done and start saying, "Hey, I can't believe I did that!" But for now, "It's easy!"

11/13/94

I found this note in one of my journals. I was always writing positive notes trying to convince myself that some day the nightmare would be over. This note was written five months before my surgery. At that time I had no clue where I would end up. I didn't even know that I'd get to have surgery or that it would ever be an option for me. My neurologist wasn't totally convinced that the seizures were not psychosomatic, and I wasn't really convinced of anything.

I always dreamed that some day I'd have my freedom back, but I began to lose hope after failing so many tests and having tried so many different medications. I began to think that the seizures would eventually kill me. No matter how positive I wanted to be, somewhere in the back of my mind I knew I was going to die from this condition if I didn't make every effort to get well.

I decided that my only hope was to put every bit of energy into being positive. I dreamed about being well all the time. I would go for long runs and pretend that I had my freedom. My mind and body were a unit when I was running. We were working together to become stronger, and we were going to win no matter what. No one could take anything away from me when I was running, not even my own neurochemical misfirings. I wasn't going to give in no matter what! Running was my escape, my freedom, my chance to dream about what I may have some day and what I could do if I had it.

So I dreamed a little each day and never told anyone. Dreaming allowed me the luxury of believing in something. Dreaming gave me a reason to live. I was the grand lecturer of "anything is possible." I truly believed and actually I still very much do believe that you should 100% follow your dreams and do nothing less than your best while doing so.

So I put every bit of energy into focusing on my goal, and staying as busy as possible so that I would never have to think about the seizures or the medication. I needed constant distractions, but it worked!

One day I'm focusing on being well, and the next day I'm waking up and I am. Okay, maybe it wasn't quite that easy, and I try not to think about it too much. But every now and then, it will hit me out of nowhere. I'll just be having a regular day and all of a sudden it will occur to me that I'm relaxed. My mind does not have to be ready for the next seizure. It will occur to me how incredibly lucky I am and how many options are open to me. I can preoccupy my mind with whatever I chose to. I have a huge freedom that only some can dream about. And then I think of how far behind I could be, I feel grateful for how far ahead I am, and I think of how much farther I'd like to go.

Σ

1. My Dedication to
the Surgical Candidate

We can't control the future, but we can make every attempt to improve the quality of our lives. Congratulations on making one of the biggest decisions a person can make with his/her life. You are a winner and deserve the very best of everything that life has to offer. If I could give you an award, it wouldn't be enough to reflect the enormous amount of credit you deserve for your strength and courage, but it would be an attempt to validate these very special qualities that you possess.

Unfortunately, there are no awards for surviving epilepsy and brain surgery. You can go to college for four years to get a bachelor's degree that will at least give you a place to put your foot in the door to start you on your way toward receiving a decent annual income.

With surviving a seizure disorder, you will be temporarily condemned to fearing a life without freedom or control. And for surviving brain surgery, you will be constantly questioned by society on your sanity and well-being. You will have to work ten times as hard to prove that you can make it, and you will have to overcome a lot of rejection in the process.

Many people will be intimidated by your ambition and your strength, and they won't know how to react to you. This is where you will really need to be strong. Often they will talk to you like you are less intelligent or weaker than they are. This can be very disheartening and can affect your healing process. Depending upon your personality and how you handle people will determine your ability to grow and to function in society in a healthy and productive manner.

I wasn't too good at dealing with rejection so I decided to isolate and write a book. Basically, this has now become my business so people have to respect me and they have to look up to me, right? Wrong! No one has to respect us ever! Of course you can kick them out of your life if they don't, or you can find a way around the situation so that everybody wins. I guess this is what I'm now working on. It seems like the really successful people have a way of working around their circumstances while being able to work with people in the process. They can also prioritize quickly, make decisions without regret, and be able to move on when something doesn't work or go their way. Not too many of us can be good at everything, but at least there's always something more to strive for.

With epilepsy, surgery is not always a cure, and sometimes not even an option or ever an option. With epilepsy, you will have to try all kinds of medication if the first one or if the first few don't work. You will go through all kinds of side effects and have to determine which ones will be the most tolerable and still give you some or if you are lucky, complete seizure control.

If the medication isn't working too well and your seizures are not showing up on an MRI, the brain scans, or the EEG, then your doctors will probably believe that your seizures are psychosomatic--that's the word they use to diagnose a physical disorder aggravated by emotional disturbances.

You will probably need to see a therapist at some point, as well. Generally, it's very difficult to get through any kind of traumatic circumstance completely on your own, but if your situation may be of a psychosomatic origin, then it will be imperative that you discuss your goals and position with a professional. I'll discuss that in Chapter Four. It's really not too bad, and I learned quite a lot about myself and other people's perspectives in the process.

Brain surgery for epilepsy is not an alternative to taking medication for seizures. Surgery is an option that may be available only if all else fails, but the results of it can be dramatically remarkable. And if I had to do it all over again, I would in a heart beat. I have written this book to help you get through the process of surgery, but I have also written it to help validate some of the feelings you may be experiencing with the seizures and to support you in your experiences along the way.

If you have chosen surgery, make sure you know the surgeon's success rate and ask to talk to his/her patients who have had the same operation that you will be having. Again, congratulations on your success thus far, and I hope what I have to offer will allow you some bit of relief in knowing that you are not alone.

Σ

2. Grand Mal Seizures

I remember the first few grand mal seizures I had were in my sleep. They were about two or three weeks apart and always left me with temporary amnesia and in fear for my life. I was in a relationship with a man that I had planned on marrying. Although we ultimately were not right for each other, Carlos was a good person and I loved him very much.

I was spending the night with Carlos when I woke up for some reason. I remember this person looking straight into my eyes and saying, "Leanne are you okay? Wake up! You just had a seizure!" This guy looked very familiar, but I wasn't sure how he fit into my life. I think he figured this out pretty quickly because he was soon asking me, "Do you know where you are? Do you know who I am? What's my name, Leanne?"

I just kept staring at him because I didn't know what else to do, and I didn't want him to know that I wasn't sure who he was. I was so scared. I didn't know what was happening or why it was happening to me. He looked awfully familiar, but I just couldn't place him. It was like I knew him but I didn't know in what capacity he fit into my life. That piece of information in my brain was not readily available.

I'm sure it was only for a few seconds, but it sure felt a lot longer. All of a sudden his name came out of my mouth, "Carlos." He was a little relieved, but I still didn't have the whole picture. Soon another man walked into the room to see what was going on. It took me a minute but I recognized Daniel, Carlos' roommate, after I saw him. My long-term memory was coming back, but I was still very confused.

19

Now someone was knocking on the front door. I thought that it was some of Daniel's friends. Daniel went to the door to let these people in. The next thing I knew, two men were coming into our bedroom and telling me to come with them to the hospital. Why was I being asked to get on a stretcher and go to a hospital in the middle of the night when all I wanted to do was to go back to sleep. My head was killing me, everyone was talking at the same time, and I was sure that I did not need this much attention.

I was very confused and very stressed, and I just wanted to go back to sleep to make this terrible nightmare go away. I was crying by this time and asking them to please just leave me alone and to let me go back to sleep. Actually, I was having a very tough time staying awake even with all of the commotion, but they were so determined to make me live out this nightmare, that I didn't know what else to do.

That night was my first ambulance ride, but not my first grand mal seizure or my last. I can't say that I remember much of that ride to the hospital, but I've been in several other ambulances since then, and I guess they are all about the same.

My understanding now is that physicians don't like the patient to sleep after generalized convulsions when the cause is undetermined. A person can have convulsions for a number of different reasons. If there is any doubt as to the cause, you will probably be taken to the emergency room for a complete evaluation before you are allowed to return home to your nice warm bed.

From the patient's perspective it is very scary, very stressful, and very humiliating. From the perspective of everyone that is taking care of us, I don't know. I have not had to experience that yet with anyone who is close to me. Once on a vacation I saw a young woman have a seizure in a line that we were standing in. She collapsed in front of us, and her family tried to save her the embarrassment by moving her out of the line. I don't know how well that worked because people were still staring and pointing at her. I can tell you that in this situation I wasn't stressed at all. But I didn't know these people, and I didn't have to take their problems home with me. I could feel for them and go on with my day.

Σ

3. How I Lived with Seizures

I don't think I ever dealt with having seizures very well. I just tried to pretend that I didn't have seizures. And when I did have them, I tried to forget about them as soon as they happened. One very important thing that I learned when I had seizures was not to panic. If I did get scared, I always found that talking myself through the fear made the outcome more bearable. This was probably one of the most important things that my therapist taught me. Don't Panic! Easier said than done, right?

I suppose the real test in living with any kind of vulnerability is knowing how not to let it take away your strength. If you tell yourself what is happening while you are having a seizure, it will psychologically set you up to handle the situation better. The best time to do this is the minute you feel that sensation that something isn't quite right. Most people I've talked to tell me that they can feel their seizures coming on. Some people have auras, some have tingling in a part of the body, some smell a strange odor, and some just have a funny feeling.

I could feel my seizures beginning with a type of aura, not unlike what some may call a deja vu. My stomach would begin having this really weird sensation in it as well. This part was actually kind of neat. But when my mind began to wander off from my body, the fun was over! This is the critical point, and how you handle this part of it will determine to a larger extent how you are going to react once the seizure is over. I would start talking myself through the situation once I felt the aura coming on.

Here is what I did to relax. I would begin with, "It's okay, Leanne, you know what is happening. You are having a seizure. It's okay, you know where you are. You know what is happening.

You can get through this. It's okay, someone will take care of you if it gets really bad. Just keep talking to yourself and don't panic! It's okay. It will be over soon. Okay, I'm in Denton. I'm laying out by the pool at my apartment, and I'm studying for a kinesiology test. I know where I am, I know who I am, and this will be over soon. Okay, I think it's over. Ahhh...... I'm okay. We did it. Everything is okay. It's over now and no one seemed to notice so I'm going to make it. It's okay, Leanne. Don't get upset. You don't need to cry, it's no big deal! It's over! You are still here, and nothing bad has happened. Okay, it's time to get back to work. Now let's see, what am I suppose to do? I better study this part because it will probably be on the test. Okay, let's read this and memorize it. Then I'll go inside and get cleaned up and feel really good that I got to be outside today and that I got my studying done. Just look at what all you did, Leanne, you are going to be so successful!"

I suppose the talking to myself (not out loud) was a way to feel that I still had some control over my life. It's also a way to keep yourself strong and not to panic. I needed strength and the only way I could get it was to convince myself I could get through the seizure and to get back to work (studying) as soon as possible. The quicker I could forget about the seizure, the stronger I felt, and the more convinced I was that indeed I would be okay.

By talking yourself through the seizure, you are trying to stay in touch with your mind. It's a weird game that you play with your brain, but it works. I'm not suggesting that we have any control over our seizures at all, but I have read other books about epilepsy by physicians who suggest this very method. I'd like to think that I created this concept out of my own ingenious survival techniques, but the truth is that I was just doing what came naturally once my therapist and I figured out how to reduce the tendency to panic.

The nice thing about having seizures (I'm a very positive person--and yes there is a nice thing) whether you are ever cured or not, you will be able to take the survival skills you learn from them and apply those skills to other aspects of your life. And if we live long enough, we'll have the opportunity to do just that.

Σ

4. The Importance of
a Good Support System

In the first edition of **Seizure Free**, this chapter was called,
"The Importance of Therapy." I've decided to rename it after going to several support groups and listening to how other people
deal with their seizures and seeing how important their friends
and family are to their healing process. The main thing is that you
have some kind of support, whether that support comes from ad-
miring those whom are more successful than you and getting motivated by their achievements, or whether that support comes from
being around people with similar problems to your own and feeling a bond that gives you strength, or whether that support comes
from a therapist, a doctor, or even your family and friends. The
main thing is to find a way to cope with the situation that you are
in. For me, it was a combination of things that mostly involved
staying busy.

Since my seizures were being questioned as psychosomatic,
I wanted to do everything possible to get well even if it meant
therapy. I did not want there to be a question about my sanity in
anyone's mind, especially my own. So I found a therapist, and I
went to her for about three years.

When I first met Kathie, she told me that her specialty was
in relationships and helping couples with relationship problems.
Well, I liked her a lot so I didn't want to have to find someone else.
I've never been too good at relationships anyway so maybe she
could kill two birds with one stone. I needed to cure my seizures,
and I figured if she knew something about relationships and had
an open mind, why couldn't she fix seizures? I pleaded with her to

take me as a new patient. I knew I could get well if I found someone I trusted with my feelings. I trusted this woman. Something about her said that she was not in this for the money. She seemed ethical, and that is what I needed.

Kathie helped me understand how to cope with my life while I had a war going on in my head. We did therapy some times three times a week. I was determined to find a cure, and I was sure that she could help me if my physicians couldn't.

We talked about everything. I talked about people I was dating, people I wanted to date, people I was upset with, and people who made me happy. I talked about my past, I talked the present, I talked about the future, and I talked about anything that I thought could be causing me to have seizures. Maybe it was something that I blocked out from my past, and now it has returned to haunt me. I talked about my family, and I talked about my friends. Mostly, though, I talked about my feelings. I had this secret wish that we'd eventually find the cause for my seizures, and we'd find a cure as a result. One day it would come pouring out of me in tears and in passion, and the seizures would disappear, magically over night.

Well, Kathie never claimed to be able to cure seizures but as long as I was there trying to deal with my problems, I didn't see any harm in trying to get me seizure free. I knew why I was upset, and I knew what I needed. I needed my life back!

So Kathie was there for me, right up to the surgery. We never did find a cure for the seizures in her office, but she offered me a lot of support and validation for my feelings. I needed a good deal of that. I had a hard time accepting reality, and she tried to comfort me in the process.

For whatever reason that my brain decided to stop working, I was willing to do anything to fix it. If the most educated people couldn't find an answer, what was I supposed to do?

You will probably need a "Kathie" in your life if your seizures are being questioned as to their origin. If not, an epilepsy support group may be more in line, and most of them are free. I admit that some times support groups can be depressing, especially if you are not a group person. However, I've seen people

24

who get a lot out of being in these groups. The Epilepsy Foundation (in America) can tell you if there is an affiliate in your area. Their number is 1-800-332-1000. If you are in another country you can check the internet for support groups closest to you. Many countries have national foundations with local affiliates for their members.

The internet system is a great place for help. There's a lot of information available and so many people who are willing to share their stories. If you'd like to remain anonymous, you can go to an epilepsy site and read what people are saying. You don't have to respond or even give out any information about yourself. This can be a nice alternative if you are not totally comfortable with telling people "your stuff." I've enjoyed meeting people through the internet.

Here is a list of some sites that I have found to be very helpful and very professional:

Massachusetts General Hospital- www.mgh.harvard.edu
and neurosurgery.mgh.harvard.edu
American Epilepsy Society- www.aesnet.org
and www.epilepsia.com
Epilepsy Foundation (of America)- www.efa.org
Epilepsy Fdn of Victoria in Australia- www.epinet.org.au
The Epilepsy Connection- www.epilepsy-connect.org

In the first edition, I also mentioned starting your own support group. There are many ways to do this even if you are not a very outgoing person. Begin by asking people at your health club, your church, your school, or your work if anyone is interested in being a part of your support group. Even if the people you ask don't have epilepsy, they will more than likely know someone who does. Just by asking them to be a part of your group will open all kinds of doors for you. If you've never done this before, I think you will be quite surprised to find the number of responses you will receive. Everyone wants to be invited to be a part of a group, even if they have no intention of joining that group.

What matters is that you get the word out that you are going to do some kind of wonderful thing for your local community. Everyone will admire your courage and that alone may invite them to be a part of your group and/or to find people for your group. If you just have thirty minutes every other week or one hour a month to meet with other people to discuss ways to deal with your living situation, that is enough! I'd suggest picking a time in your schedule that is most convenient for you, since you are going to need energy to get other people excited about your idea!

It's really important to sound excited and to be really positive about starting a group, any kind of group! Being positive creates a sense in other people's minds that you know something they don't! They will want to find out what you know, and they will want to have some of your positive energy rub off on them. Being excited about your group makes others interested in your ideas and interested in you.

After you have told your friends and family about your support group, decide on a time to meet, and then schedule your meeting somewhere fun, like at a good restaurant, but not an expensive one! This will get everyone in a good mood to open up and to join in the conversation.

Get names and numbers of volunteer drivers for your event. And list those people on the flyer that you will hand out announcing the first meeting. Make sure everyone has a ride, and find rides for people who can't drive. Try to meet at an off hour, like 4:00 p.m. in the evening on a Saturday or Sunday to avoid the crowds.

If you decide to meet at someone's home instead, pick the hour most convenient for the host, and ask everyone to bring something, like a pot luck dinner. Ask everyone to contribute one positive event that has happened to them recently, or one event related to epilepsy that caused a problem and how they handled the situation. The idea is for everyone to learn something in the process of supporting the group. Learning together will give everyone confidence in addition to offering support. And bringing confidence to the group will get everyone to focus on the solutions, not just the problems! Good Luck!

Σ

5. I Was Embarrassed
Because I Had Seizures

I can't figure out why people have a problem with accepting epilepsy. According to statistics, one in one hundred people have epilepsy, but in my mind that does not matter. Epilepsy is still socially unacceptable, and people still treat us like it's a disease.

When I was first diagnosed with epilepsy, I didn't tell anyone because I didn't want to believe it myself. As time went on, the seizures got worse. I felt like I was forced into needing to tell people, and I certainly didn't like that either. I knew that I had to open up if I wanted to increase my chances of survival when I had seizures in public, but I hated every minute of it.

To have to tell an instructor or a student or a co-worker or anyone that I had epilepsy was a nightmare. I felt like I was giving in by just saying the word epilepsy. I felt like I was disclosing the most secret part of my entire life and then hoping to God that no one would take advantage of my vulnerability. I hated it! I hated how it made me feel, I hated how it might make me look, and I hated the word! I hated every aspect of it, and I hated that it took away a part of my youth!

I felt controlled by needing to tell people about it. I always had this fear that once they found out, my life would end. They'd treat me like I was sick and unable to do the things that they did. I felt like once they knew about it that I had to work ten times as hard to prove myself so that I didn't get that label attached to me of being weaker than anyone else or being "disabled." So I did work ten times harder! I worked my butt off! I wasn't going to stay home and give up, I'd rather have been dead! I had a job, I was going to school, and I ran, a lot!

Most of the time when I told people, it was not really that big of a deal to them. I tried to choose wisely when I did tell someone. But every now and then, I'd get a weird reaction. I can laugh about it now because it really is funny. But when you are feeling the pain of having to divulge a secret piece of your life that you are not very proud of, it's not funny when the person reacts in a hostile or an indifferent way.

I remember a certain math instructor that was not too keen on the idea of having someone with epilepsy in her classroom. It was the first day of class, and we just sat down to begin. She went through the syllabus and told us about her rules. I was sure that this was not going to be a very fun teacher at this point. She was very serious, and she meant business.

After an hour and a half of listening to the instructor, the class was dismissed. I waited for a few of the students to leave so that no one else would hear me when I told her the terrible news. I walked over to the door just as she was beginning to leave. I remember looking into her eyes and searching for the strength, "I have to tell you something. I kind of have epilepsy, but it's okay!" She looked at me rather oddly and wasn't too sure what to say. I could tell that she probably had no experience in dealing with this kind of situation as she was very insensitive to my needs. She rebutted with, "Well, what does that mean?" She was very nervous at this point, but she was also very harsh. She paused and then said, "You're not going to have a seizure in my classroom, are you?" She sounded as if I had just offended her, so I told her that I'd try not to have a seizure in her classroom. I wasn't quite sure what she was so upset about. She could go home and be well! I couldn't!

I went home that day and tried not to think about it. I knew I would have more than enough of her just being in her classroom. I guess I could have responded with, "Yes, I am going to have a seizure in your class, and I'm going to have it at the most inconvenient time so that your lecture will be interrupted and you won't have a clue what to do about it. I'm going to have as many seizures as possible this semester, but I'm going to save them all up for your classroom. I think you need a little experience in sensitivity and this is going to be your chance to learn. If you don't pass the test, you will be fired. I get to be well, and you will lose your job!"

Too bad we can't make those kind of deals in the real world, huh? Too bad we don't get to choose our disabilities? And too bad that we don't get to play those kind of games with life?

Looking back on my life, I shouldn't have had a reason to be feeling like I needed to prove anything. I was already doing more than the average person was anyway, and certainly doing a lot more than the people I was feeling insecure around.

If you feel like the people around you are treating you like you're not as good as them, I'd move on. I suppose that's just common sense but sometimes when we are caught up in our issues, it's hard to see through the anger and the pain. It's almost easier to continue trying to prove we are good enough, than to move on or to just say, "I don't need this kind of treatment in my life!" Finding people who believe in you from the beginning is a much better way of living. You'll go much further in life, and your real friends won't be threatened by your success.

Σ

6. My Scariest Seizure: *I Thought I Was Dying*

Most of my seizures were complex partials that would occasionally turn into grand mal seizures. I think one of the scariest seizures I ever had was in the women's locker room at college. I was on my way to an instructor's office to turn in a report. I felt like I was having a deja vu so I went into the locker room to sit down for a minute. I knew what was coming, but I didn't know how bad it was going to be. There were other people around as well. One girl asked, "Are you okay?" I told her that I was having a seizure, but I would be fine. She told me that her sister was epileptic and that she was used to taking care of her. After that, I don't remember what happened. We were talking one minute, and the next minute I was entering hell.

I didn't know where I was, but I knew that my brain was not with my body. I could feel my arms starting to shake, and I didn't know how to stop them. Someone was talking to me and telling me to relax. "It's okay. Just relax. I've got you. Come on now, try to relax."

I didn't know how to communicate with the voice and the more I heard it, the more scared I became. Where was the voice coming from? Where am I, and how do I get out of here? What is going on in my mind? How do I escape? Give me an answer! If this is hell, let me die!

I wanted it to end, but I didn't know what was happening. If I was dying, why did it have to take so long? Why can't I hurry up and die? Please let me die! Make this end, now!

I could feel spit coming out of my mouth, but I didn't know

how to stop it. I think I could feel someone trying to hold me, but I didn't know how to reach this person because I didn't know where I was. All I knew was that I wanted it to hurry up and end. Why did it have to take so long?

I could feel my arms and shoulders shaking and my body falling forward but again there was nothing I could do about it. I didn't know where I was or how to escape. I could hear that voice again, "Just let go, it'll be okay!" I couldn't communicate with the voice and I've never wanted more in my life to die. I didn't know where my brain was or where my body was or even who I was. If I was supposed to die, why couldn't I? I just wanted it to end and I didn't care how.

I started feeling sick. Too many sensations were happening all at once. I could now feel slobber drooling from the side of my mouth, and it was causing me to choke but I couldn't do anything about it. I couldn't see anything, either. Maybe my eyelids were flickering but I still couldn't see anything. I wanted to open my eyes, but I couldn't. I wanted most to have contact with the outside world, but I couldn't reach it.

The next thing I remember, there were these paramedics standing around me. I remembered being hunched over and spitting up and these people telling me to relax and to let go. I was somehow coming to my senses. I was waking up and feeling very embarrassed for what my body was doing. I was sobbing and scared to death. Where had I just been? And why was I here?

The paramedics were telling me to calm down. They kept saying, "You just had a seizure. Now calm down!" Oh sure, it was no big deal to them. I could have just died, and I'm not sure that I want to live knowing this has just happened and knowing that it can happen again. I don't know that I want to be here, and they are telling me to calm down. What the hell is wrong with these people?

That is what I am thinking now that I relive the situation. At that time, however, I was too traumatized to be angry. Anger would have taken too much energy. Here is what I said to them, "I'm just so tired of this happening. I just want it to end!" I know that's

32

what I said because that is what I always said. Just thinking about it makes me cry. They say that crying is good for you, but I don't know. Some things are just better left alone. Some things just don't need to be relived, you know?

I know now that seizures put everyone under stress, even the people that are trying to take care of us. I was never really able to see that until this last year. I was always so caught up in the seizures being something that I had to fight alone that I wasn't able to see how my life was affecting those around me. I wasn't able to see how my living in denial scared the hell out of everyone else. I'm sorry for that because I never meant to put anyone under stress. I was trying to deal with the situation the best way that I knew how. I was trying to do as much as I could so I'd have something to look back on and something good to remember. And it worked!

Four years ago I was having brain surgery. Today I'm remembering the "good old days." That's pretty funny isn't it? I'm finally far enough away that I can look back and laugh! I can look back and remember the people who were there for me, and I can remember how special I felt to have them in my life. I see the world a little differently now, and I can laugh and cry at the same time when I think of my past. I'm sounding really old, aren't I? I had a birthday not too long ago, and I think that's what this is all about.

I'm sure everyone must look back at the hard times in their lives and feel lucky for what they have now. It must be an aging process that we all have to go through. It's probably just a way of coming to terms with our pasts.

Σ

7. Medication

Depending upon the type of medication you are on, it is very important to check with your physician before you take any other medicine or herbal supplements. I've decided to include herbs in this section as I've heard a few people saying that herbs may help them. And they may. However, a lot of medication can alter the effectiveness of anticonvulsants, and if you are like me, you want to know if the seizure medicine is working and you want to know how well it is working.

You've probably already been told that drinking alcohol may decrease the effectiveness of your seizure medication while the medication can increase the side effects of the alcohol. I like to remind people just in case they haven't heard this yet. The way I see it our bodies can survive an entire lifetime without a drop of alcohol, so why risk it? It just seems like our brains are already so delicate, why add another potential problem to the already existing nightmare?

I'll tell you what I do remember about mixing medicine, and I didn't even know this would be a problem. In the winter months, I get sinus headaches like most everyone else in the world. I used to take a nasal decongestant that contained acetaminophen (Tylenol) and a drug called pseudoephedrine HCl. The pseudoephedrine HCl is in a lot of over-the-counter sinus medications and works really well for the temporary relief of nasal and sinus congestion. Unfortunately, it also increased my seizure activity. The problem was that everything else mixed with the already intoxicating side effects of the seizure medicine put me to sleep. I couldn't afford to be any more intoxicated, and this pseudoephedrine HCl kind of gave me a little more boost. The point is that I took it some times any way because I got tired of being stopped-up and having sinus headaches. I found out later that my doctor could prescribe a preventative that could keep my sinus pathways open during those winter months. The one I used was called Nasacort. It is a spray that you use everyday in each nostril to decrease inflammation of the mucous membrane. It seemed to be quite effective for me, and it didn't increase my seizure activity after using it. If you are having the same problem I was, I'm sure your doctor wouldn't mind ordering something for you, too.

Some anticonvulsants need to be taken continuously in order to be effective, while others require only a single dose a day. The single dose a day is easy to remember if you always take it at the same time and in the same place. Keep a single dose of your medication in a weekly or a monthly pillbox. You can pick up a pillbox at your local pharmacy or grocery store for just a few dollars. This pillbox could save your life.

After seizures, we are a little confused and experience some short-term memory problems. If you keep your pillbox by the kitchen or bathroom sink, you can always check it to see if you forgot to take your medicine for that day. You will then know what to do, or you will call your neurologist's office and the nurse or someone on duty will be able to tell you what to do.

If the medication you are on requires that you take several doses a day, I suggest that you get a weekly pillbox and carry it with you everywhere. Buy a wristwatch that has an alarm feature on it. The one I used could be set to go off as often as I needed it to. With Lamictal I was taking 700mg a day, and I only weighed 115 pounds. I would set my watch to go off every four hours so I could take small doses of medicine throughout the day. After almost every dose, I would get a little dizzy for the first few minutes. I tried to always have granola bars and Nutrigrain bars with me. I would usually have a snack when I took my meds. This would kind of offset the effects of the medication. I learned how to eat small amounts of food all day long. Actually if I had ever eaten to be full, I would have been very fat. I was always hungry, but tried to ignore it until I absolutely couldn't stand it any longer. Trying to keep my body in good shape was a good part of what gave me self-confidence to deal with the seizures.

I am a big advocate of exercise. I started running as way to feel good in the mornings before going to work. It was probably the first positive habit I ever created. I'll tell you how it began. I was tired of staying out late drinking with my friends when I knew I needed to be at work the next morning. I'd wake up feeling bad, and then arrive for my first appointment feeling groggy from the night before. I just didn't see that lifestyle going anywhere, and I was very conscientious about my work. So I decided I'd have to change some of my habits if I wanted to do better in this world.

I started out by doing a walking/jogging routine a couple of mornings a week just to see how it would feel. And it felt pretty good! Each time became a little easier and each time felt better. It seemed like those days turned into weeks and weeks turned into months and months turned into years, and before long I had established a real healthy habit. Somehow it became a part of my life. It was like making your bed in the morning. You just do it!

But when I started jogging, I was also a smoker. I was having such a hard time breathing while exercising that I decided to cut back on the cigarettes. I figured I'd see how I felt without the cigarettes and then I'd go from there.

That was thirteen years ago. I'm still running, I haven't touched a cigarette since then, and I no longer drink. Basically I came to the decision that drinking is just not too good for some of us, and smoking is good for no one! So I decided to change these habits. The good news is that I had given up drinking about two years preceding my epilepsy diagnosis so that was one less thing to worry about.

Σ

8. *Outpatient Procedures:*

Magnetic Resonance Imaging (MRI)

Most people diagnosed with epilepsy will need to have an MRI done at some point in their treatment. The MRI allows your physician to distinguish the fine details of structures in your brain. With this information, your neurologist and the radiologist can determine if there are any abnormal structures present. If you lucked-out and this is your first one, maybe I can give you some advice. Try to think about something relaxing when you go in for your appointment.

Your technician will have you put on a robe and then lie on your back on an examining table. You will be wheeled into this big white tunnel-looking thing. You will need to be very still because this machine is going to be taking pictures of your brain. While doing so, it will sound scary and seem weird, but just keep thinking about whatever allows you to feel relaxed. Personally, I tried to pretend that I was at the beach. This always works for me, but you may have a better idea. Go with it, and Good Luck!

Some hospitals are now using open MRI's and you may ask if one is available in your area. With the open MRI, your body remains outside of the tunnel. People claim that they feel less claustrophobic in the open MRI by comparison to the traditional closed MRI. Either way you'll do fine, but remember to think of something that relaxes you!

Computerized Axial Tomography (CAT)

The CAT scan is a lot like the MRI in that you will be lying on an examining table and a large white dome will be taking pictures of your brain. The x-rays are detected by a scanner and fed into a computer to come up with a cross-sectional "map" of your brain.

A contrast dye may be injected into a vein in your arm and used to make the soft tissues in your brain more visible. This way your doctor can see changes in tissue density in your brain. This will help to rule out a possible brain tumor or major artery disease.

Supposedly, the contrast dye has side effects of nausea and feeling flushed. I can't lie! When I had the CAT scan done, they used the contrast dye on me, and I did not like it one bit. I remember lying down and being told that the shot was not going to hurt. Well, the shot itself didn't hurt, but the minute that the dye went into my vein, I thought my brain was going to explode. It felt like this pressure was building up in my head, and I didn't know how to stop it.

I don't want to scare you because it's really not that bad after it's over. That's a good one, isn't it? Nothing's that bad once it's over! Okay you may have a headache for awhile but nothing that a little Tylenol can't cure. I'm sure you'll do fine! You may want to ask your neurologist if he/she can leave out the contrast dye, though. I don't know if this would be an option, but it's worth the inquiry.

Positron Emission Transaxial Tomography (PETT)

The PETT scan shows the rate at which biochemicals are metabolized by your tissues. The results for this test may tell your physician if you have dead tissue in your brain or if a tumor is growing.

The PETT scan is painless and requires that you lay down on an examining table and be wheeled into a large hollow cylinder. A natural body substance, such as glucose, will be injected into a vein in your arm. This substance will help distribute an image of the tissues in your brain for the scanner. Your doctor can then identify any biochemical changes by observing a series of these images. Don't worry! The substance in this process that is going into your body is nothing like the contrast dye used in the CAT scan. It will probably feel like water going into your vein, and you will forget about it. After doing the other tests, this one will be a piece of cake. Good Luck!

Magnetoencephalography (MEG)

The MEG is still relatively new and was not used on me, but I can tell you that it is supposed to be painless. The MEG measures magnetic fields in the brain much like the EEG measures electric fields. With the MEG, small detectors are applied to the surface of the scalp. These detectors gather information to determine seizure origin and can even be helpful in mapping certain brain functions, such as speech and motor movement. According to Dr. Bruce, "It is likely that this test will be used increasingly over the next few years and may help decrease the need to perform invasive monitoring with electrodes."

Single Photon Emission Computed Tomography (SPECT)

This test measures the amount of blood flow to the smaller areas of the brain and involves two procedures. The first part of the test is a base line measurement called the "interictal" study. The second part of the test is called the "ictal" study and looks at changes in the brain at the onset of the seizure. Usually there is an increase of local blood flow during this time. The idea is to find the increase in local blood flow at the onset of the seizure and then to determine its origin.

You will be given an intravenous injection of a short-lasting radioactive isotope and your brain will be scanned with a two-headed camera. I am told that this procedure is also painless and involves minimal noise. When I had surgery, I did not need to have this test but the painless part sounds like a pretty good deal! Dr. Bruce says that the actual scan can be done when the seizure is over since the radioactive drug remains in the brain for an hour or more after the isotope is given. This benefit of the SPECT is something that makes it particularly valuable in the study of epilepsy.

Σ

9. My Worst Seizure
Experience: The Aftermath

After one particular bad episode of seizures, I was having a lot of problems for about a week and a half. On this particular occasion, I must have had two or three grand mals in a row. My brain liked to do that. It didn't start out that way, but as the situation progressed, the seizures would last longer, they'd get stronger, they'd come in clusters, and over time they'd become less predictable. At first I just had the grand mals in my sleep so I could still justify driving. But one day that would change, too!

So the aftermath was sometimes worse than the seizure itself. Remember when I told you about my scariest seizure in Chapter Six? Well, the weird part was that I recovered quite quickly. I took notes back then because I was trying to find a cure. According to my notes, after leaving the hospital, my memory was at 75%, or "fairly good." And by evening my memory was back to 100%. I know that part of the reason I recovered so quickly was that I did not get a load-up dose of Dilantin in the emergency room (ER). For some reason, my doctor did not order the load-up dose that time like he usually did.

For those of you who don't know, a load-up dose of medication is sometimes given to us when we've had a bad seizure. For me the load-up dose was 700mg of Dilantin. A standard daily dose of Dilantin is around 300mg for a person with epilepsy. Basically, they just want to give you a little extra protection before leaving the hospital. Yes, you will be confused and depressed for a while from the seizure and from the extra medication, in that order, but the alternative isn't so great. If you don't get some kind of extra protection into your bloodstream, and your brain decides to start seizing again, you will be in even worse shape and maybe a lot of danger. So this is just one more thing that we have to get used to and adjusting to it is very hard on a person and hard on the people around us.

There are other aspects to having people take care of you as well. You will be getting bills in the mail from everyone. These people include the attending physicians in the ER, the hospital itself, and the company who provides the ambulance service. We can't just be left in peace to forget about the seizures. We have to pay lot of money for people to take care of us when we 'd rather just be left alone. Maybe this sounds a little ungrateful, and I mean no disrespect. Paramedics have to work very hard, and they have a tough job. But some times I wondered how necessary all of that treatment was. People have seizures, and it sucks! What is the hospital staff going to do besides give us extra medication. Not that that isn't good enough, but some times that leaves us in worse shape.

They can't make us well! And we still have to go home to face another day of potential seizure problems anyway. Tomorrow you will have to work twice as hard to make the money you will need to pay for all of that wonderful treatment you received in the hospital. And the stress of knowing this is enough to create another seizure, right? Do you think this is going through their minds when they are hauling us off to the hospital? Well, you get the point!

Now before I get too carried away, I want to give society a little credit here. Although I often felt patronized by having to go the hospital, I never had anything stolen. Every single time, my backpack and all of its contents would end up in the ER with me and would be given back to me when I checked out. I usually fell asleep in the ambulance so never remembered the rides. So for those lone heroes who looked out for my well-being when I was too tired to do so--THANK YOU! You never went unnoticed but you may not have received a "thank you" on site. You were always very much appreciated, but probably didn't get to find out. So after this really bad episode of seizures, I was having a lot of trouble recovering. I found out later that I was given some Ativan in the ambulance. Ativan is a drug that is used to pull a person out of convulsions. It worked well for me, but it also left me groggy and very depressed for a couple of days. Add that to a load-up dose of Dilantin in the ER and then the normal recovery time from the grand mal seizures, and you are going to be really messed up for awhile. I'm not saying its anyone's fault! Nobody wants us to be sick, but that much medication in your body is just not a fun experience.

I felt like I had too many things to recover from with this particular event. It's kind of making me nauseated just thinking about it. I don't want to be a baby, but I'm going to take a break and finish this in a minute. I'm really feeling sick!

Okay, I'm back! The nice part about writing is that I can take a break whenever I need to and it doesn't have to interrupt your reading. What a great deal for both of us, huh?

So after that experience with the seizures and the medication, I was having a really hard time recovering. I couldn't find the words I needed to express my thoughts, and I was having problems with my short-term memory. I was even stuttering quite a bit and could barely follow the lectures in class. It was so embarrassing but I tried to hide it as much as possible.

I think being in school added to the stress when I was having seizures, but for the most part, it allowed me to feel a real since of accomplishment. It allowed me to feel like I was still smart, and my brain was still working okay.

I was really angry with my neurologist for ordering that much medication to be put into my body. His name was Dr. Leroy. He also happens to be one of the best in the business, but at that moment, I was seriously questioning his intentions.

On my follow-up appointment, only a few days after that episode, I had a serious talk with him. I was mad, confused, and nervous. I couldn't find the words I needed to express my thoughts and that made it even worse. This person has just done this crappy thing to me and now I have to fend for myself. I was pretty sure the odds were in his favor, but I didn't care. I was mad and hurt! "What's the idea of.......ahm....giving me...me....so many drugs? You know what that does to me! I can't concentrate...[I was sobbing].....I can't...can't even talk! You ... you can't do this to me!" He was less than thrilled by my attempt to stand up for myself. He just leaned over confidently and said, "Listen, Leanne, if I think your life is in danger, I will do whatever I have to, to save you!"

I don't think he liked my situation any more than I did, but he certainly did not want me questioning his methods of treatment on this day. Under different circumstances, we'd talk about treatment and the like, and just about anything. He has always been a good listener. He takes his work seriously, and he is good. But when it comes to life, he is open to just about any conversation. He doesn't get offended easily. In fact, I kind of miss talking with him.

I remember the first couple of years after surgery when I told him I was thinking about going into medicine, the first words out of his mouth were, "Well, you are certainly bright enough. And you have empathy for people. Why not? You'd be a good doctor!" I almost fell over! That's the best compliment I've ever had, and I will always remember. From that day forward, I decided that the successful people on this planet believe in themselves so they have the ability to believe in others. And you know some times that's all it takes!

Σ

10. The Stages of Testing
for Brain Surgery

Most epilepsy units have a way of classifying their procedures into some kind of system. At Southwest Medical Center and at Medical City in Dallas, the stages of testing for surgery are classified into three phases. Phase I refers to the EEG video monitoring with scalp electrodes. This procedure is a noninvasive method that records your brain waves while you are being videotaped in the hospital. The idea is to have seizures while staying at the hospital so your neurologist can see how your body is reacting to the seizure, as well as to how your brain waves are responding. This may take from one day to two weeks or even longer, depending upon when you have seizures and if they show up on your EEG. I will tell you exactly what to expect during this procedure and how to plan for it in the next chapter.

Once you have completed your Phase I monitoring, you may or may not need to go in for the Phase II monitoring. The Phase II monitoring refers to the EEG video monitoring with depth electrodes, subdural strips, or subdural grids. This procedure is done when your doctors can't find an exact focal point for your seizures. They want to be absolutely sure before removing a part of your brain.

With the depth electrodes, two holes are drilled through the top of your skull and long thin electrodes are placed down into your brain. You will be monitored all over again just like in Phase I, only this time the electrodes should give your neurologist a focal point for your seizures.

With the strips it's basically the same idea, only the surgery for this procedure is a little different. The surgeon drills a hole through the skull and slides a numbered strip between your skull and your brain. The strip sits on top of your brain over the suspicious area. One strip may have ten different numbered electrodes in one single row.

The surgeon may place a long strip through a hole in the skull, or several strips through two or three holes in the skull. If a larger area needs to be monitored, the surgeon may need to open a part of the skull--this is called a craniotomy--and place a subdural grid, as required. The grid is composed of the same substance as the strips, only it consists of several rows of numbered electrodes so it can cover a much larger area. Once the grid is placed, the skull is put back on, the scalp is sewn up, and the patient is ready for monitoring.

Each electrode within the strip or the grid has a specific number. When you start having seizures, your neurologist will be able to look at your EEG and match the numbers on the strip or the grid to your abnormal brain waves. This information is given to the surgeon so he/she knows exactly where to go to operate. It's really a very neat system.

Fortunately, I did not have to go through the Phase II monitoring, but the operation for these procedures can take one and a half to three hours, depending upon your surgery. Once you are ready for monitoring, you will be in the hospital until you have seizures just like in the Phase I stage. It all depends on when your brain decides to have seizures.

Once a focal point is found, your surgeon will remove the depth electrodes, the grids, or the strips and then be able to remove the abnormal brain tissue if everyone decides this is the best treatment for you. "Everyone" refers to you, your family, your surgeon, your neurologist, your radiologist, and anyone else who becomes involved.

Phase III refers to the actual brain surgery itself. Again, this is only one system for classification, and each hospital has its own way for classifying their procedures. I just wanted to include this chapter to give you an idea of what to expect.

Σ

11. EEG Video Monitoring:
What to Expect

I decided that I wanted more from life than just a way to try to deal with having seizures. That was a great start, but why couldn't I have more? I wanted to be well, and I wanted my life back! So the next step was to do an EEG Video Monitoring.

The idea with this monitoring is to stay overnight in the hospital and to try to have seizures. A video camera will be hanging from the ceiling or attached to the wall at the end of the bed. This camera is going to be taping your every move. When you do have a seizure, your neurologist will have something on tape to look at to see how your body is responding to the seizure. This information may help determine what side of your brain the seizures are coming from and is combined with the EEG results to get a more accurate diagnosis of your situation.

Once your neurologist says that you can do the monitoring, there are some things that you need to consider. You will need to be available for an extended amount of time so that you can stay in the hospital long enough to have seizures. You will also want a friend or close relative there twenty-four hours a day. If you can get your friends to take turns being there, that will allow you to be covered at all times.

You should take someone that you trust with your life. This person should spend the night in the hospital with you and be available to answer questions from the hospital staff. I'm sure that your physician will agree with this. Most units today have an extra chair or sometimes even a small cot where a family member can stay in the room with you.

When you arrive at the hospital, someone will take you to your room and begin placing electrodes on your head. Your technician will first apply a type of solvent with a cotton swab to each location on your scalp. He/she will rub each spot to remove oil and debris that could loosen the electrode once they begin the monitoring.

Because the electrodes have to be secure, your technician will use a type of glue to hold them in place. This part doesn't really hurt, but it can be rather uncomfortable. Just keep thinking about how successful you are for being chosen to be monitored. You have come a long way and gone through a lot of tests to get to be in this monitoring unit, and you deserve to know what is going on with your brain. This is your opportunity to find out!

Once your electrodes are in place, your nurse will want to run some intravenous (IV) lines into your arms. This is just one of those standard hospital procedures that needs to be done so that your vitals can be checked regularly. One IV line will be for fluids that they want you to have. Mostly this is a way to keep you well-hydrated during your hospital stay. Another line will be used on your other arm with a heplock attached. This is just a precautionary measure in case they need to give you medication or something else. You will also have electrodes attached to your chest and wrist, monitoring your heart and pulse rates. It sounds scary, doesn't it? Really it's not that bad.

When I did my monitoring, I was so scared of having the seizures that I was glad I had all of those other things to keep my mind preoccupied. You can think about what kind of neat fluids are going into your body and how many calories that will add up to. Isn't that silly! I was worried I'd get fat from lying in bed and being hooked up to bags of liquid (calories) running into my body. I was worried that I'd be stuck in a room without anything to work on or anything to do. I took homework with me just in case I had time to study, and my brain wasn't seizing. Okay, maybe I'm a little weird, but I loved my life. I loved school, I loved cutting hair, and I loved running. The problem was I didn't like what came with my life--epilepsy!

Nurses and technicians will be coming into your room and asking you questions about your medication and your treatment and all sorts of stuff. It will be very hard to answer their questions because, hopefully, you will be having seizures. This is where your friend or family member comes in. When they get to the technical stuff that friend will have the information they need. Also, you may want water or a soft drink or something else. A friend can run to a coke machine or to a restaurant to get you real food. If you are having seizures, it may be difficult to get to the bathroom by yourself, this is really where you will want that close person to be there for you.

If your neurologist wants to keep you on medication for some reason, keep a notepad by your bed and write down every time you take medicine, even if the nurse is giving it to you. It's a very good idea to keep these notes yourself, just in case there is a misunderstanding somewhere along the way. If you are having seizures, make sure that the person with you is keeping good notes for you.

Another way to protect yourself is to take a mini-cassette-recorder with you. This way if any of the attending physicians need to tell you anything, you can start the record button and listen to it later after you've completely recovered from the seizures and from your hospital stay. There won't be any miscommunication if it is on a recorder, and you will have the information you need when you are able to concentrate better.

There may be a TV and a VCR in your room. More than likely, you will have both. If there's a movie that you've been wanting to see, take it with you. Now is your chance. Of course if things go as planned, you will be having seizures so you won't remember much of the movie anyway. But take some video-tapes just in case. I think my sister, Kay, was more excited about the videos than I was. She loves movies! She couldn't wait to show me the movies that she had picked out for us. I think we ended up watching stand-up comics most of the time, and she and my friend, Wendy, did the movie watching when I was sleeping or trying to do homework.

They will want you to stay awake for as long as possible, trying to stress your brain into having a seizure. This was the hardest part for me. I remember feeling really nauseated from drinking coffee and from being up all night. It is difficult to get any kind of physical release because you are stuck, for the most part, in a bed. You don't really get to have much activity. I was used to running about twenty to thirty miles a week, and lying around in a bed waiting to have seizures was not on my list of things to do for any given day.

I'll tell you why exercise was so important to me. I hated feeling intoxicated. The exercise gave me a way to release the tranquillizing effects of the medication. Exercising made me feel like my body was fighting the drugs, and it allowed my brain to take a break from the mental stress of the whole situation. Being stuck in a hospital was very, very stressful for me. There's no place to go to get away! You are just stuck there with people telling you what to do and how to do it, and everyone watching you to see if and when you are going to have a seizure.

I just kept thinking about my clients and the girls at work. I kept thinking about how the sooner I could get this done with, the quicker I could get back to my schedule and feel like my life was making a difference in the world.

The night they made me stay awake was a real nightmare. They kept me on meds for the first three days because I was too scared to come off of them. So staying awake was the next option and it was really hard to do being on my seizure medication. I cried most of the night. Kay and Wendy stayed with me. They seemed to be a pretty good team to have on my side. They'd hold me and make me laugh, and all sorts of stuff. They took turns watching me and taking naps. I was the only one who wasn't supposed to be sleeping. Kay reminded me, "Sleep deprivation can be a torture treatment. You know they used it as a form of torture in concentration camps and on prisoners of war when they want to get secret information out of them!" I was relieved, "Goo (that was her family nickname), I'm glad you told me that! I remember hearing about how they tortured prisoners. That sounds familiar. That would explain why I feel like I'm entering hell!" She empathized, "Lee, I just wanted you to know that you are not crazy. I am just validating your pain! So don't you feel better, now?" I guess that did make me feel better. She always has a way with words and she always knew how to validate the problem and then to just let it go. I don't think they liked it any more than I did, but we all knew what had to be done.

When my monitoring was done, the electrodes on my head were attached to wires that were all connected to these cables that ran into this big machine. This meant that I needed to wear a shirt or a gown that opened up in the front. I took some button-down shirts with me because I wanted something from my home. Wearing a hospital gown the entire time did not sound too appealing to me, and I suspect you may feel the same way. Also take some cotton slip-on shorts because people will be coming in and out of your room and you probably won't want to feel too exposed.

My stay in the hospital was not too productive. They tried making me hyperventilate, they tried sleep deprivation, and they even pulled me off my medication on the fourth day of my stay, but nothing seemed to work too well. My brain had just decided not to have any seizures while I was there.

Actually, I do remember feeling a few light auras but apparently they were not big enough to be recognized on the EEG as anything significant. Everyone was beginning to wonder about me and to seriously question my condition. But I'll tell you what, I was a very active person back then, and lying in a bed was not one of my normal routines.

The medical world is now getting caught up with the idea that being in a hospital is a different kind of place than the real world for the rest of us. And for the patients, the stresses of the hospital are quite different than the stresses in the real world, and the monitoring results may be affected by these differences.

On the seventh day I went home off medication, and thinking I had a serious psychological problem. I was becoming desperate and I needed an answer. Unfortunately, we were not able to get that answer in the monitoring unit. But when I got home, I felt great in every other way. Physically I had so much energy because I had been in bed for so long, but also because I had been off meds for at least five whole days.

When I left the hospital I was as confused as their staff, but Dr. Leroy agreed to leaving me off meds to see what would happen. If I did have a seizure I was to call him immediately and to go right back to the hospital. They'd get me all hooked up again so we could try to get something on tape and on the EEG. That certainly sounded like a reasonable plan to me. So that's what we did!

I felt great! I could think clearly and my body was full of energy. The last time I felt this good was four years ago before the seizures started and before I had started taking medication. It was almost like I was on drugs because I felt so good. You know that feeling you get after having the flu? Well, you know that feeling just as you are recovering, like you are so strong again? That feeling of "AHH...I feel so much better!" It was a little like that except 100 times better with a clear head as well. I can't even tell you how good it was. It's like your thoughts are processing much quicker and your body feels so strong and the world seems less complicated. Everything is so clear!

Two days after being home and back to work, everything fell apart. Wendy was staying with me. I think she kind of knew this wasn't going to last. She had a way of knowing things like that. Actually everyone was telling me to be careful, but I kind of wanted to pretend that I was well.

So we were just sitting there having a conversation about the world, and discussing where we might be in ten years from now. Well, you can guess what happened. One minute we are talking, and the next minute I'm waking up with a paramedic telling me to come with him to the hospital.

You know it's so scary when you have a grand mal seizure because you lose time. You lose pieces of information, and you lose entire days. It's like everyone has to keep telling you what is happening, what day it is, and where you are. You can lose pieces of information even as someone is talking to you. Generally, I would fade in and out of sleep and each time I would start to wake up, they would have to tell me the whole story all over again. I hated it, but my memory would just be shot for awhile. It's like your brain doesn't know how to get in touch with the moment. It is just too exhausted to remember, and trying to remember takes a lot of energy.

There's this thing in your mind that tells you the sooner you can remember everything, the more secure you will feel knowing that your brain will be okay. This has got to be very hard for the people around us. I can't imagine having to tell someone something over and over again. It's like I had all of this anxiety that my memory was going to be lost forever. I don't know if this is a fear for you, but that was one of my biggest fears. I suppose that's also why I was so ready for brain surgery. I didn't want to take any more risks with the grand mals. It always felt like my brain was being so damaged, and I had no clue how to protect it.

On this day, I actually got to have two ambulance rides. The first one took me to the local hospital in Denton where I lived. The second ambulance took me to Parkland Hospital where we would start the monitoring all over again.

So the nurse and EEG technician got me all hooked up again in the monitoring unit, and we waited. As we waited, I found out something. I had two grand mal seizures in a row at my apartment before the ambulance picked me up. When I got into the ambulance, I had another one. Apparently they were concerned for my well-being so they gave me a shot of Ativan to stop the convulsions. Normally this would have been exactly the right thing to do, but the Ativan was awfully strong. Trying to monitor me now with so much medication in my body wasn't of much use.

After three days, they sent me home again with more useless information and a bill for five thousand dollars. We tried, but it didn't work. I know Dr. Leroy must have felt bad about the situation, but I'm also quite sure that I felt a whole lot worse about it.

I would need to get back to work to try to recover some of

the money I'd need to pay everyone for their time and their care. Looking back on this, I think we should have been a little more patient. I probably should have just stayed in the hospital until I had seizures and then worried about the money part of it later. But it's always easier to see things in hindsight, isn't it?

Σ

12. EEG Digitrace:
One More Attempt

After leaving the monitoring unit, I wasn't too sure what to think. I got to be home for two whole days off of medication before the nightmare returned. I thought I had my freedom back and it felt so good for those two days. I got to go to work and be able to think really clearly for one whole day, and Wendy and I got to have a lot of fun on that second day, until the grand mal started.

Well, Dr. Leroy hadn't quite given up on me, yet. He mentioned doing something called a Digitrace System. This is a system that monitors your seizures at home. Basically it is a small portable EEG unit. He felt like this might be a good alternative since I was such an active person. Of course I agreed with him.

We started this procedure about two weeks after the Parkland experience. This particular procedure involves going into the hospital to get scalp electrodes hooked on and then taking a fanny pack with you that contains a portable EEG system. You go home and wait to have a seizure and when you start having one, you push this little button on the EEG unit. This starts recording your brain waves. When you've got enough abnormal brain wave activity recorded, you take the unit back to the hospital and they retrieve the information from this unit. At night, you have to recharge the battery by keeping it plugged into an outlet in your home.

Actually, it's kind of a lot of trouble because you also have to go back to the hospital if any of your scalp electrodes come loose. It seemed like mine were always coming loose so I needed to get someone to take me to the hospital each day. When I was in the monitoring unit at the hospital, a nurse would usually come in to re-glue the electrodes about twice a day, a convenience you won't have at home.

I remember walking to school after I started this digitrace monitoring. I just stuck to my schedule and pretended like everything was normal. I put a hat on my head over the electrodes and tucked the cables under my shirt. I also said a little prayer on my way. I figured it wouldn't hurt anything to ask God for a little extra help. So I prayed that I'd make it to class and that I'd get home okay without having any seizures. If I could just get through the day and to make it home, that would be a major accomplishment. I could have the seizures later. That's what I was hoping for.

On my walk home, I felt really successful. I sat through an entire class, and no one even noticed that I was attached to a cable line. What a challenge that was! I made it to class, I got through the day, and I even got home without anyone noticing anything was wrong. I guess I was feeling pretty strong!

I only had a few auras that night while we did this digitrace unit and again they were not big enough to be detected on the graph. We should have been more patient, but I didn't want to go into debt waiting to get well. If you have the opportunity to do any kind of monitoring, I'd highly advise being patient. Don't worry about the money or school or work or anything. Find out what is wrong with you first!

I wish someone would have told me that, but maybe no one thought about it. So you'll have time to make all the money in the world, but you've got to get your brain working first, or if nothing else, at least find out what is wrong with it!

Σ

13. A Psychosomatic Disorder

It would be two more years before I got to do the monitoring again. During this time, I was dedicated to my therapy. I was even more determined to find an answer now that it looked like my seizures could be of a psychological origin. At this point, I didn't care what was wrong, I just wanted to know what it was so that we'd be able to figure out how to fix the problem, or at least be able to reduce my anxiety about it.

When I was first diagnosed with epilepsy, an in office EEG was done on my brain, and my brain waves were diagnosed as "epileptiform in character." A psychological condition was not even a consideration.

Over time, however, my EEG was no longer showing any obvious abnormal brain wave activity. The MRI only showed minimal scar tissue in my temporal region, and even that was questionable.

So now the only hope I had was to discover what my mental problem was so that I would stop having seizures. I was willing to do anything. The way I saw it, if I could solve the problem by continuing with therapy, why not try? It would be a lot less risky than brain surgery, a whole lot less expensive, and a whole lot easier on everyone involved.

A part of me kind of liked the idea that the seizures could be psychological. That meant I had the power to solve the problem. It also meant I had an amazing ability with my mind, even if that power was working against me. If I could solve this problem, I could do just about anything.

So I pretty much became obsessed with getting well. I was also kind of mad that nothing was working. I didn't want to be a failure, and this whole experience was doing absolutely nothing good for my ego.

I knew I had to find an answer, but I didn't know that by believing the problem was psychosomatic that I'd be setting myself up for failure. By allowing the patient to think the problem has a psychological origin puts the responsibility back on that person. Unfortunately, it also makes the patient feel guilty when he/she is already doing everything possible to get well. I felt like I was causing a lot of trouble because I couldn't just deal with my issues in a healthy way. I had to inconvenience everybody else by having seizures!

I didn't want people to revolve around me because I had a medical problem and/or a mental illness. I wanted people around me because I was such a neat person and because they saw my potential, or maybe even just because they liked me. But to be around me so they could pity me was not my idea of good company. That wasn't going to make me stronger, and it wasn't going to get me well.

Σ

14. I No Longer
Wanted to Live

Regardless of what I wanted, I still felt like my life was going downhill and there was nothing I could do to stop it. I tried to be positive, but I was gradually giving up. I just did not see that there was much of a future living with a seizure disorder that couldn't be fixed or found. What I mean is that if they could have at least found abnormal brain waves, I could justify the problem and reduce the responsibility that I had to take for it. I could have said that it was not my fault, and maybe allowed myself to have some distance from the problem. Perhaps then, I would have learned to accept it and deal with it. But I didn't see that as an option from where I stood.

I felt like I was losing everything in my life, my relationships, my independence, my hope, my energy, my sanity, my security, and my life. And it was all my fault! I didn't know what was wrong with me or how to get my life back. I loved doing hair and taking care of my clients, but even that was becoming more difficult. School gave me a way to maintain some of my confidence, but it just wasn't enough. And after the seizures, school was so difficult that I'd lose whatever confidence I had worked so hard to gain in the first place.

I had been on and off of Tegretal, Dilantin, Depakote, Tranxene, Lamictal, Neurontin, and Felbatal, and nothing seemed to work with much success. Each medication has its own special side effects that include everything from feeling sick, tired, confused, nauseated, intoxicated, and bloated, to irritable, feverish, and nervous twenty-four hours a day. And I was still having about fifteen complex partial seizures a month, along with an occasional ambulance ride to the ER for convulsions. The grand mals seemed to be coming more often and usually came in threes. Nothing was working, and my life was falling apart in the process! I was just running out of energy!

I went through all of my emotions with Kathie, and we discussed a lot of things from my past. I just kept hoping for something, anything! Maybe because I was molested as a child? Maybe because of something else that happened that I wasn't aware of? Maybe because I was angry or stressed? Maybe it was my diet? Maybe it was from the caffeine in my tea? Maybe it was something I was doing or thinking that caused me to have seizures? Maybe, maybe, maybe! How about, maybe nothing! How about, I was angry and stressed because I was having seizures. How about, I drank ice tea and water to keep me awake because I was on so much medication? How about, a lot of children are molested, but that doesn't mean they are going to start having seizures over it! How about, nothing is making sense any more! How about, I check out!

Well here it goes--I no longer wanted to live! I was fighting a battle and I didn't even know who the enemy was. There was no way to escape because the seizures followed me everywhere I went. There was no "safe" place!

I didn't want to be remembered for having a seizure disorder. I wanted to be remembered as someone who cared about people and who wanted to make a difference. I wanted to be remembered as a positive person who worked hard and who enjoyed life. I wanted to be remembered for my contributions, not for my illness. I did not want to be remembered as a person who was dying. Epilepsy may have taken away my life, but it wasn't going to take away dignity!

I decided there was only one way to end this war. From my night stand drawer, I pulled out a pistol. I put the bullets in the chamber and cocked the gun. If I could just end everything peacefully and not hurt anyone else, I'm sure my friends and family would forgive me. Wouldn't it have been more selfish of them to expect me to live when I was so miserable? They won't have to feel bad for me because it will be over! If I can no longer have hope, I can no longer live!

Growing up, my father taught us about guns so we knew exactly what the rules were. At this point, I no longer care!

I put the barrel in my mouth and my finger on the trigger. I remember pulling my finger and the trigger moving, slightly. I then told myself to finish pulling the trigger, and the nightmare would be over. I would be at peace once and for all. No more fighting, no more crying, no more anger! The war would be over, and I would be free!

Σ

15. Maybe I Wasn't
a Complete Failure

Before I could finish pulling the trigger, I looked down at my stomach and noticed something. After all these years, I had finally become the person I thought I had always wanted to be. My stomach was beautiful, not an once of fat on it anywhere. I never had a very good body growing up, and I always felt ugly. For the last two years of my life, my running had become an obsession to be in perfect shape. I had the most perfect body a person could have. I couldn't be a failure, I looked too good. I was very depressed and didn't feel like I could make other people happy because I was too unhappy with myself. But maybe I wasn't a complete failure.

At this point, I let go of the trigger and threw the gun on the bed. I began weeping terribly and wasn't too sure what to think. I cried all the rest of the night and never told anyone except Kathie.

I have decided to go ahead and publish this because I think it might save someone else's life. I think you also know that this is not about how good I thought I looked. This was about convincing myself I had a reason to be here. The people who may have needed me, I didn't feel like I could help any longer. So I still needed to know in some way that I was not a failure. If I couldn't make my brain work, I could at least feel good about my body.

Σ

16. Life Is About
What We Do For Others

Today I can't imagine thinking that my body being perfect has anything to do with my self worth as a person. My body is just a part of who I am, and it does not have to be perfect. In good shape would be nice, but perfect, nahhh...!

Today I'm more focused on how much of a difference I can make. I'd like to know that what I've done matters and that it mattered to someone in particular. I'd like to know that my existence made a difference in someone's life in a very positive way. I'd also like to know that in some way I made a difference to the world. Yeah, that's a pretty big wish to request, but why not? I don't really have anything else to do. The way I see it, if you can't dream, you can't do much! I suppose if I really believed that I was so wonderful, I wouldn't need to make a difference. I would just go on my way and pretend this never happened. But for some reason, I can't do that!

Σ

17. The Half-Marathon:
My Longest Run

For the last two years I had been involved off and on in drug protocol studies. It sounded scary at first, until I realized what a great deal it was. I had to track my seizures and report side effects to my research nurse, but then I also got my medication for free. The drug protocols I did were for lamotragine and felbamate. Lamotragine was the last medication that I was on before surgery. The side effects weren't too bad until I had to be on higher doses, but even then I still had about fifteen complex seizures a month along with the occasional grand mals.

The felbamate, I was taking toward the end of '93. I don't think that I stayed on felbamate for more than three or four months because the nausea and the nervousness were side effects that I couldn't handle too well. In addition, I was still having seizures.

I do remember one thing very well about felbamate--I ran the White Rock Lake Half-Marathon on it. When the race started, I was ready to go but felt really nauseated. I kept thinking that I was going to have to stop and throw up but kept telling myself to keep going. After half a mile, it got worse. My stomach felt like it was in all kinds of knots and the nausea was not going away.

I trained six months for this race, and I wasn't going to stop running. I tried to focus on other stuff around me. I tried to think about the music--I always carry a cassette player. I thought about the different instruments and how they sounded. I also tried to focus on my surroundings. I studied the trees, the leaves, the sounds of other runners' footsteps, the wind on my face, the pebbles and rocks along the side of the path--anything to keep my mind off of my stomach. I kept telling myself to keep going, no matter what! Before long I was coming up on mile four, and the nausea was beginning to subside. As I began to feel better, my speed was picking up, too. After those first few miles, I had it made. The next few miles were easy. I was on my way now. I was becoming lost in the music, and my mind was enjoying the ride. With running, once I got warmed up and established a comfortable pace, it was very easy to get lost in the music. It's like you become so free and so at peace with your environment that you forget about your problems.

I thought about everything when I was running. I thought about the conversations I'd have with people I was close to and the conversations I'd like to have if the opportunity ever presented itself. I thought about people I wanted to date and how I could get them interested in me. I thought about my family, my friends, and the people I cared about. But I also thought about how my life used to be. I thought about how I used to believe anything was possible, and that I was immortal. I thought about how some day I'd have my freedom back. I thought about what it would feel like not to have seizures and not to be on medication all the time. And then I thought about how lucky I was for having legs that worked so well, how lucky I was that I could run.

When I started training for this run, I told myself the only goal I had was to complete the actual race itself. If I did finish it, it would be neat to do so within two hours. I didn't want to put too much stress on myself just in case something went wrong. My training distances were between ten and twelve miles, and the half-marathon is 13.2 miles. I figured I'd do fine.

I was coming up on mile thirteen, I felt absolutely great, and I even had enough energy to do a little sprint to the finish line. I always liked to save a little energy for the end. It also seemed to confuse the people around me and that was kind of fun.

That was one race I'll never forget. And guess what! I finished in just under two hours. That translates to roughly nine minutes and ten seconds per mile. Okay, so can't I brag a little? I'm not saying that I'm an athlete or anything, but I think I did pretty good for a thirty-year old woman.

Σ

18. *I've Just Been Given Hope*

The date was January of '95, and it was time for my regular checkup with Dr. Leroy. This particular appointment turned out to be quite a good one. For some reason, he asked me again if I would consider brain surgery. This was like asking me if I wanted my life back.

The last EEG video monitoring I did was two years ago, and the only diagnosis we had to go on was a possible psychosomatic seizure disorder. The seizures were getting worse, and I wanted to know more.

The day after my appointment, I got a message on my answering machine saying that I needed to call his office because there may be an abnormality in my brain that will show up on the original MRI X-rays. I felt like I was dreaming. I remember the first time that we did the monitoring at Parkland. No one could agree that there was anything wrong with my brain other than a little scar tissue, but with a normal EEG, that was not a significant finding.

So why did he change his mind all of a sudden? And why now? The one thing I did know was that I wanted to get those X-rays over to his office as soon as possible. I started calling people right away to find someone to give me a ride. One of Kay's friends said she would take me. Anyway, we went to Parkland to get the X-rays to deliver to his office that very day.

It's so exciting picking up X-rays of your brain. In the car, I pulled the X-rays out to see if we could find the damaged part. There was a little black spot on the film. "Hey, look, here it is!

This is where the seizures are coming from! What do you think? This is the part that's causing me so many problems. Maybe they can just remove it. Won't that be great! They can just take it out and send me home!" We had it all figured out!

I couldn't wait to show Dr. Leroy my ingenuity. I kind of wanted to show off when I got there by pointing out the damaged part before he had a chance to go over it with me. Boy was he going to be impressed!

Well, it didn't exactly work like that. When I arrived at his office, he was ready for me (in between patients, of course). He took the X-rays out of my hand and fastened one of them up onto the X-ray light.

Before I had a chance to say anything, he looked it over and said, "Okay, do you see this area here?" Yeah I could see that area, but why didn't he want to discuss the damaged part? "Well if you look closely at it, you can see a variation in shade. Can you see that?" I wasn't too sure what I was looking at, so I just kind of said, "Sure!"

He pointed at that same area on some more of the X-rays. Then he said, "That's the suspicious area!" I don't know, but it didn't look quite as obvious to me as it did to him. It seemed like that "black dot" that I had picked out was a lot more blatant than what he had discovered.

Unfortunately that black dot that I found was nothing. It wasn't even in my brain at all! It was something that just got on the film in the processing of it. Well, I guess you figured out that Dr. Leroy wasn't going to get to experience my ingenuity on that day!

So he showed me the damaged area, and we made an appointment for me to do another monitoring a month and a half later. We would also need to set up an appointment for a PETT scan in between this time. Everything would be done at Medical City in Dallas where his new office was.

I was so excited I could hardly wait! I just felt like I was having this wonderful dream. I wanted the dream to last forever, but I wasn't too sure that it was going to. I kept thinking I'd wake up eventually. But for some reason, I didn't!

I had a month and a half to get ready for my monitoring so I decided to tell a couple of my instructors that I wouldn't be in class for a few days. I had one instructor that I really liked. I remember that I had told her some where along the way that I had epilepsy, and she was so cool. She didn't look at me weird or tell me not to have seizures in her class, or anything. She just asked me how she could help and if there was anything she needed to do for me. I gave her Dr. Leroy's number and asked her to call him if she ever saw me having a grand mal seizure.

A couple of weeks after that, I was in her office visiting with her, and I noticed that Leroy's phone number was on her wall. I can't remember if I put it there or if she did, but the fact that it was still there meant a lot to me. She actually kept his number up after that for quite some time. I always felt kind of special when I went by to see her. I don't think anyone had ever done anything like that for me before.

Her name was Dr. Goode, and she would eventually become my advisor. I don't think she ever really knew how important she was to me, but I felt very special to have her in my life.

I told her about the monitoring and how I'd miss a couple of her classes. She was so understanding about the whole thing. I think she kind of knew that I wanted to do well in school, and that it bothered me to have to take off like that. I wouldn't have missed her class for anything! She loved teaching! She had this wonderful way of accepting people and understanding her students. She would come into the class and get everybody motivated and involved in her lecture. She never had that "I'm so important because I'm a professor" attitude. She just really loved what she did, and it showed!

So I didn't want to miss class, but I knew I had to. This was my big chance to find out what was wrong with my brain. I had a whole month and a half to think about what Leroy had told me. This damaged area in my brain could have been a number of things. It could have been scar tissue, a type of inflammation, or even a possible small brain tumor.

That brain tumor-thing didn't sound so good. The other stuff I was used to hearing so I wasn't too worried, until he mentioned a "possible small brain tumor." Then I began to worry about it. I tried to pretend like I didn't hear that part, but it was hard. I broke down in one of Dr. Goode's classes, and she asked me if I wanted to share this information with the class. No Way! I was ready to run as far away as I could, but she was only trying to help. She didn't understand that I didn't want this to be a group activity. I already felt weird enough.

I was only thirty-one years old and not ready to have a brain tumor. I think the brain tumor was just mentioned as a worst case scenario. Dr. Leroy had never talked about this before so I just kept trying to forget that I heard that part. Besides, we wouldn't know until after surgery anyway, so thinking about it wasn't going to do me any good.

Σ

19. EEG Video Monitoring:
My Second Chance

I had been through this procedure before so I had a pretty good idea of what to expect. I knew two things for sure: first, I wanted to get this activity over with as soon as possible, and second, I wanted to have a lot of seizures so that someone could find something abnormal on my EEG and tell me that I wasn't crazy.

I decided if I took myself off medication the night before the monitoring, I would increase my chances of having seizures when I got to the hospital. If I took myself off meds too soon, I'd risk the chance of getting to do the monitoring by having the seizures too soon. My life could be in serious danger, as well.

So I decided not to take my nightly dose of Lamictal. This would be safe enough, and yet still a very practical way to handle the situation. This would surely increase my chances of having a seizure, but I'd be leaving to the hospital in the morning so that would give me just enough time to get there before my brain went haywire.

I also didn't sleep. If I didn't get at least eight hours of sleep a night, I would have at least one seizure the next day. So I stayed awake for as long as I could that night. I probably got a couple of hours of sleep, but for someone with seizures that is as good as no sleep at all. So I was ready!

Kay dropped me off at the hospital on her way to work and Mom met us there. My mother was always good about volunteering her time for these events, but I never liked to impose on my family. I decided this time would be a good time to let her volun-

75

teer as I may not remember much, if my plan was going to work as I had hoped it would.

And I don't remember much of my stay. They must have put the electrodes on after I got to the hospital because all I know is that I got to the hospital just in time to lay down in a nice warm bed and to fall asleep. The next thing I remember is waking up with my mother beside me and a couple of nurses telling me that I just had three complex partial seizures and two grand mals and that I could go home. I couldn't believe it! Nothing had ever been that easy!

It was true! Dr. Leroy stopped by to release me and to give me some of the best news I've ever heard. "Hey kiddo, you did it! Your seizures were recorded on the EEG, and it confirms the MRI report. We now have enough information for you to have surgery!" He couldn't have meant me. I knew I had seizures because of how I felt, but I wasn't sure if he was really being serious about the surgery part. Maybe he just said that to see how I'd react. I was tired and disoriented and not even sure of what day it was or how long I had been in the hospital.

"You mean this is it? We're done? You found something wrong with my brain, and we can fix it?" It just seemed too easy, I guess. Six years of seizures and medication, and a couple of years of therapy and now I can have an operation just like that?

Everything seemed too good to be true. But there was still more to do as Leroy explained, "Well, I will need to have a board meeting with the hospital if you decide you want to have the surgery."

What could he have been talking about. I thought he was the boss. After all, it was his epilepsy unit. He was "the doctor" for studying patients with epilepsy. I wanted more details about this board meeting. I was a hairdresser and never had to consult with anyone except my clients when making decisions. This medical world was a completely different concept. Maybe I was just naive, but I was kind of under the impression that doctors had all of this control and independence. They got to make big decisions with people's lives, and then they got to be paid a lot of money as their reward for getting to do so.

It doesn't exactly work like that, as most of us now know! I would soon forget about the complicated world of medicine and its politics as I will discuss later in Chapter Thirty-One.

I kind of wanted to know who was going to be getting to make this decision with my life, other than Dr. Leroy. So I asked, "Who exactly attends this board meeting?" He told me, "Let's see, there will be three neurosurgeons, five neurologists, two radiologists, and a few other staff members. I will need to convince them that you are a good candidate for this type of surgery. I will need to tell them why this will help you." I was really shocked, that many people just to get me well.

Today it makes me feel incredibly special, but back then, I had very low self-esteem and didn't want to take up people's time. I felt like my illness was causing all of these problems, and it made me feel very uncomfortable. If I had known that doctors liked sitting around talking about that kind of stuff, I'd probably have felt differently.

I can tell you that if I had to have surgery today, I'd get the very best surgeon, and he or she better have a good team to work with. I'd also like to have a surgeon with empathy and a good personality. I've been spoiled by the latter and understand that not all surgeons are charming and personable, so I'd settle for a great surgical track record and good follow-up treatment.

Anyway, I was pretty excited about this new diagnosis. While Leroy was scheduling his board meeting, I would need to schedule an appointment for a neuropsychological test.

Σ

20. The Neuropsychological Information

This procedure is done after your neurologist and his/her assisting physicians decide that your EEG, MRI, CAT scan, and PETT scan are all showing similar evidence for your diagnosis. In my case, the seizures were coming from my right hippocampus. I would need to have this part of my brain removed as well as the right, lateral side of my temporal lobe. The neuropsyche information would determine if the left side of my brain would be able to compensate for the parts on the right that were to be removed.

It sounds scary when you put it down on paper, doesn't it? But if you are having seizures and your medication keeps you intoxicated most of the time, the word "surgery" sounds more like a miracle cure. Getting a part of your brain removed doesn't sound nearly as bad as living with seizures the rest of your life and being on medication that doesn't work too well. So if you are considering surgery for yourself or someone you know, this is the point where I have to tell you to hang in there. We are almost through with "the tests."

When I arrived for my appointment, I was taken to a room and given a lot of paper work to do. This part was the easiest. I was in school and used to this kind of treatment. There were some oral tests as well as mechanical. A woman would read a story to me, and I had to repeat it back to her. I also had to repeat long lists of numbers in forward and reverse order. That was easy, too!

Then came the hard part. I started to cry on this one because I was so scared. I was blindfolded and told to place objects in their proper location-- a circle block goes into a circle hole, a square block goes into a square hole, etc. It sounds simple enough, right? It's not! You can't see, and one hand has to be tied behind your back. The woman placed an object in my hand and told me to put it into the correct hole somewhere on the table.

So I'm trying to feel the object with just my hand, and I couldn't tell what it was. I knew it was a block, but I didn't know its shape. It felt like it could be oval or maybe oblong or maybe some kind of variation of these shapes. I really didn't know, and I couldn't find the place for it on the board.

It's kind of like you have to feel the object and then set it down so you can feel the hole in the board to know where to place the object. I just couldn't figure it out. Then I tried fitting the object into the hole and that didn't work any better. I don't know why it was so difficult. I started to cry after the third of fourth block because I was tired of taking tests and I was so frustrated with myself for not being able to accomplish such a simple task. I felt totally incompetent and began to worry about the condition of my brain. What did this mean? Have I lost my sensation of touch and spatial relationship? Why was it so difficult?

This deal is an all day event by the way, and it is very stressful. I'll tell you why. A test of any sort creates anxiety, probably a healthy anxiety, but none the less an anxiety. When that test is your shot at getting your life back, there's a lot to think about, and there is a lot of pressure on you to perform well. With school if I didn't do well, I got a bad grade. I could always discredit a bad grade by saying the test was too biased or I didn't study enough. I could still make it up in the end if I did well the rest of the semester.

With this neuropsyche test, my life was on the line. This was my final destination! If I failed this test, it was over! I may never get this chance again. A lot of important people have worked really hard to get me here, and if I fail, not only is my life over, but I will have let all of these people down. What will I do then?

I had to do well, but that was not a good way to look at it. The problem is that this is not a test that we have any control over. It's not like you can study for it, or practice and become better. It's just a way of determining if both sides of your brain are functioning okay. If they remove the damaged area on the right side, will the left side take over so that you won't be left with any deficits? There was no way to study or prepare, I just had to hope my brain did what it was supposed to.

Σ

21. Brain Surgery:
Making the Decision

Once you get your results back from the neuropsychological information, you will be on your way. If your brain doesn't do what it's supposed to on this test, again it's not your fault. After all, if we could control our brains, we wouldn't be having seizures, right? I just wanted to be sure to throw that part in just in case things don't go as planned.

And if things don't go as planned maybe you weren't supposed to have brain surgery for some reason, and there are still other options available for you. I wanted to include this special note so that you don't give up. There's always hope somewhere. You may ask your doctor if you are a candidate for a vagal nerve stimulator (VNS). They are implanting quite a few of these now, and a fair amount of people who haven't had good seizure control with medication seem to be doing much better with the VNS.

I know they recommend the VNS for various types of seizure problems, and especially for people who may not be candidates for brain surgery. Today if I had a choice of getting the VNS, I would probably try it before removing a part of my brain. The way I see it, why not? My surgery was very successful and yes, like I said I would do it again if I had to, but it doesn't hurt anything to be conservative when it comes to removing a part, or parts, of your brain. I think you get the point!

I will tell you that I've had the opportunity to observe a VNS implant, and it is quite interesting. The stimulator is placed just under the surface of the lateral border of the major pectoral muscle. Leads, attached to the generator, travel from a program-mable chip to the vagus nerve on the left side of the neck. The leads wrap around the nerve and stimulate the nerve by sending it programmed signals from the chip. Stimulating this nerve is thought to increase seizure threshold and abort the seizure. It may be an option worth looking into.

Anyway, if things do go as planned and you are ready to have brain surgery, you will need to be strong for your family and friends, that is, the ones that are there for you. Your close relatives and friends will be rather worried, even if they are being support-ive. Unfortunately for them, this is the hardest part. I didn't un-derstand this before now because I was too consumed in my own survival plan. Now that I've had a little distance from the situa-tion, I can see that it was very hard for them to let go of me and to say, "If this is what is best for you, then you have to do it!" That seemed more like a guilt trip before, but not now. They were do-ing all they could to keep from crying. The fear of losing you is overwhelming to them, but they have to hide that if they care about you.

This is how it worked for me. I had just been given the opportunity to get my life back. I've never worked harder for any-thing in my life. If you are my friend, you are going to be excited for me. It seems very obvious and clear, doesn't it? Well, it did to me at that time. But looking back I can see how it may have been a little difficult for outsiders to get excited for me. Their perspec-tive was entirely different from mine.

Here's an example of what can happen. When I was plan-ning to go into the hospital for my second monitoring, I was tak-ing a physiology lab, along with some other classes. I would need to get incompletes in these classes.

When I told my lab instructor that I was going into the hos-pital, she tried to give me a lecture on the dangers of operating on one's brain. She was more concerned with giving me a lecture on life, than listening to my story. I was totally humiliated! I was so excited, I had worked so hard, and she couldn't wait to give me a lecture. Could anybody be more selfish? She was more concerned with giving me what little information she knew about the brain from her physiology teachings, than to be sensitive enough to acknowledge my position.

I felt like my judgment was being questioned. She was not even a doctor, and she was giving me a lecture on something she obviously knew very little about. I didn't need any criticism or judgment calls. I'm quite certain that I was old enough and intelligent enough to make decisions that risked my own life. Most of risking my life I had very little control over. I risked my life every time I showed up for class! I risked my life every time I went to sleep, and I risked my life if I didn't get enough sleep. Everyday of my life was a risk! Now someone has just given me some of the best news I could have--I may have the option to live a better quality of life. The last thing that I needed was negative feedback!

Okay maybe I still have some issues! But I needed to include this story for those of you who may experience a similar communication problem with someone. Now maybe I can recap this experience for you:

I'm all excited about my test results (to get to have brain surgery) and can't wait to tell someone. This someone has not had to live the last six years of her life looking for an answer to a life-threatening illness. This someone is in a position of authority and sees it her responsibility to deliver information to those less fortunate than herself. This person is trying to get a degree that will allow her to go out into the real world and practice law. She sees herself as superior to her students and feels a need to impress her students with this wonderful information that she has worked so hard to obtain. A student is excited about getting to have brain surgery. The instructor can see that obviously this student doesn't know what she's getting herself into and sees it as her responsibility to educate the student.

Well, I don't doubt that this recap of the experience is a better way to look at this conversation. I can see a lot of things differently now. I don't want to forget the anger or the pain, though, or I won't be able to give you my real feelings and you may not be able to relate to me. One of the goals after all in writing this book is to validate some of your feelings. So I will continue to give you both of my perspectives, then and now, and maybe we can see eye to eye.

So it's not every day that a person sounds excited about getting to have brain surgery. I think for the rest of the world surgery is seen as a negative alternative to solving one's problems. Most people end up in surgery by accident, not by choice. Most people don't go through years of testing to find out what is wrong with them. Most people don't go through years of medication and experimental drugs trying to find something to control a serious problem. And most people can't imagine thinking of surgery, especially brain surgery, as a "wonderful option."

These differences in perspective for us create a lot of communication problems. The only advice I can offer is to understand that there are some very real differences in our perspectives, and those differences can cause us to fight with people, to feel misunderstood, and to give up on the world. I know it doesn't seem quite fair that the vulnerable person has to do the adjusting to society when everyone else is in a better place to do the adjusting, but somehow that's how it always has to be. The minorities of the world have to be stronger if they want to make it. The world is not going to adjust to us, so we kind of have to learn to adjust to the world. If we can't adjust, we can't make it!

Am I sounding like that instructor that needed to give me a lecture? Okay, I apologize. But if you can learn to adjust to the world's weirdness, you will be the successful one. I'm saying this to remind myself, but I'm also saying it to validate your position. It's hard to laugh at a situation when you feel like others are laughing at you, but you have to try! In the end, you will come out looking like the hero and the other guy will just look stupid for giving up on you!

With my temporal lobectomy, there was an 80% success rate for patients becoming seizure free after surgery. There was another 50% chance that I could come off medication if I was seizure free after surgery. As far as I was concerned, that was good enough. I worked for a very long time and awfully hard at trying to find an answer. When I was told that I could also have the surgery, I was more than ready to try it.

Although I was ready, there were some risks involved. My surgeon, Dr. Bruce, said there was a 2-3% chance that I could have a stroke during the operation. He explained this further by telling me how I could have that stroke. If he cut this particular artery in my brain while he was operating on me, that stroke would occur. The way I see it, anyone confident enough to be that honest has to know what he is doing. He didn't try to cover it up or anything. He just came right out and told me. Pretty cool, huh? Well, I thought so, especially since he knew I was taping him.

There were some other risks as well. I may have some short-term memory problems, and I may have trouble with language skills or vocabulary following the operation. As far as I was concerned, my short-term memory wasn't working too well anyway, so I didn't see this as much of a loss. The language skills didn't seem critical enough to worry about, and the vocabulary I could work on. The other risks are too minimal to mention. Those risks will be mentioned on the papers you fill out before surgery. Those papers just say that you won't sue anyone if something goes wrong, so long as they do their best to save you. You either sign the papers or forget about the surgery. In other words if the surgeon accidentally cuts that artery, you will forgive him/her, so long as everything was done to protect your health and your well-being.

With seizures there are never any guarantees. I didn't feel like the alternative to surgery, living with seizures the rest of my life on medication that didn't work too well, was any better than the risks involved in having surgery. In my opinion, surgery was the only answer for me.

Σ

22. Brain Surgery: Scheduling and Pre-admitting

On March 20, 1995, exactly six years since my first grand mal seizure, I was on the phone scheduling my appointment for brain surgery. This next part I have to tell you about because I think you will see the humor in it. When I called to make the appointment, the receptionist asked me when a good time for me to come in would be. We agreed that April 12th would work out just fine. When I asked her what time I needed to be there, she hesitated and then said, "Well you are his first appointment that day." I interjected, "You mean he does more than one of these surgeries in one day?" You have to realize that this was a very monumental thing for me. I couldn't imagine that there were that many more people waiting in line to have brain surgery. Anyway, here's her response, "Well, yours is relatively simple surgery!"

I think I was more shocked than offended. If this was such a simple procedure, why didn't we do it a long time ago when the seizures started getting bad? If this was such a simple procedure, why did I have to go through so many tests and so much mental anguish just to get there? I think in a way I felt like she had just minimized everything I had worked so hard for. I did not need to know that this was no big deal for anyone else. It was a very big deal for me!

Anyway, since it was such "simple surgery," now I could relax! Actually, I was too excited to worry about what she had to say or what anyone had to say. I was going to get to be a pioneer! I was going to be a part of something that people would be talking about forever...if it worked!

Everything went by so quickly that all I could think about was what it might feel like to be seizure free again. I just wanted to hold on to that feeling forever.

After you schedule your appointment for surgery, you will want to contact the admitting department at the hospital to let them know when you will be arriving. You will have a lot of paperwork to fill out when you get there even if you are only having the "simple surgery" procedure.

The admitting department will let you come in a day or two before your surgery date. On this day, they will want a down payment and/or your insurance information. They will also want you to sign a bunch of papers that say you won't sue anyone if anything goes wrong. I'm sure you know that this is just standard hospital policy. Just make sure that in those papers everything looks consistent with what your physicians have told you. If you have any questions, have them call your neurologist's office or your surgeon's office. Let their receptionists or nurses clear everything up. They are good at that, and they have to do it all the time anyway.

You may want to consider the risk of losing blood during your operation. With my temporal lobectomy the odds were very low, but I still wanted some of my blood on hold just in case there was an unexpected emergency.

Your neurologist can contact the blood bank in or near the hospital and order a withdrawal. You will need to have this done about seven to ten days before your surgery date, but don't quote me on that. They are very specific about the timing of removing your blood and keeping it preserved. It can't be done too soon or too late. So make sure you ask your doctor about this at least three weeks in advance of your operation.

Σ

23. The Night Before Surgery

The night before surgery, I couldn't sleep. I stayed at Kay's house and slept in her bed with her. Kay had fallen asleep. As I was lying next to Kay in bed I remembered thinking how we used to spend the night in each other's rooms as kids. We used to play with each other's hair and tell jokes. It was like we had our own private slumber party. Now I have just made the biggest decision of my life, and I may never get to see this person again.

She is my only sister! Does she know how much I love her? Does she know how much I'd miss her? Who would be my confidante? Who would take care of her?

I started to feel a little selfish. I'm risking my life because I want a better one. Where does this leave my family and friends? I never expected anyone to take care of me, but I couldn't go on in the shape that I was in for much longer and pretend to be happy. I always saw unhappy people as unsuccessful people, and I certainly didn't want to be unsuccessful. I also didn't want to be a failure, and I didn't want to lose. So does this make me selfish? If they really love me, they will have to let me take this risk, and they will have to understand.

Looking back, I can't say that I was scared. I may have been feeling a little selfish, but I was too excited to feel fear. On a much smaller scale, it's kind of like the night before you are going to learn how to snow ski, or water ski, or ride a horse for the first time. It's like the night before you travel to a foreign country for the first time. It's like being a kid and knowing that tomorrow is Christmas and you are going to get to open all of your gifts.

You are not thinking about what you won't get, you just want to see what you did get. I was too excited to acknowledge fear.

I must have dozed off right before dawn because I remembered thinking that it was about time for the sun to come up just before the alarm went off. I was out of bed and dressed in just a few minutes. There was no need to waste time since I wasn't allowed to drink or eat anything after midnight anyway. This meant no morning coffee or anything!

On this very special morning, I could sacrifice my coffee, my peanut butter and banana sandwich, and my glass of water that I always had before my morning run. These parts of my morning routine would have to be put on hold until after surgery.

I did take my morning dose of seizure medicine as prescribed, and hoped that it would be enough to keep me protected from any seizures before the operation. I wanted to remember everything from checking into the hospital to being wheeled into the operating room. I was hoping that my brain would not short-circuit and make me forget this part of my life. This was the biggest day of my life, and I didn't want to miss anything!

Ode To a Bad Relationship

Part I.   Sometimes
we become so content
with the environment
we live in,
that no matter how much pain,
anguish, and instability
that exist within it,
it is still much better
than the fear of change.
I now believe
that I have some concept
of a battered woman
in a bad relationship.

A relationship begins
with the thrill of passion
and Euphoria continues to follow.
All of your dreams come true,
until one day your marriage
becomes a nightmare.
The person you once loved
with such admiration
has just become a monster.
But you have become
so used to this monster
that you don't know
what life would be like
without it.

One day you are finally
given the chance
to leave that monster
and to go back to the good life
you once had,
but with the knowledge
you have acquired
from this relationship.

93

*Once again all of your dreams
have come true,
and your excitement
is so overwhelming
that you still can't believe
it's true.
You must be dreaming.*

*And when that actual day
comes to move out
and start your new life,
you hesitate
and question your judgment.
What you once knew was
100% the best thing for you
has now become your greatest fear.*

*What will you do on your own?
How will you start over?
Who will be there for you
when you get home?
No matter how bad
the relationship was,
you still knew what to expect
and who would be waiting for you.
But now what?
Where will you go?*

*On your way out the door,
you smile,
knowing that deep in your heart
this new life will be better
than anything you ever had before.
However, on the surface,
you still question your judgment
and wonder how you will make it
through your fear
on the way to your new life.*

Part II.   *I once believed*
that all my dreams
had come true.
My career became
my all consuming passion.
Then one day
something changed my life,
And being diagnosed
with epilepsy
brought my world
crashing down around me.
What happened to my career
and where did the passion
for life go?

I was so in control of my life.
How could anything
take it away from me?
Where could I go
and how could I get home,
when the seizures followed me
everywhere I went?
No matter how far I ran,
they seemed to always outrun me.

Then one day
after accepting the epilepsy,
the chance came
that I could change my life.
Once again,
all of a sudden,
all of my dreams had come true.
The feelings
were so overwhelming
that I jumped for joy,
and then cried for fear
that I was only dreaming.
I had the chance
to get my good life back,
but with the survival skills
I had acquired along the way
from the seizures.
How could this be true?

95

Then that day came
when I scheduled
my appointment
for brain surgery.
I began to question
my judgment
and wondered if what I
once thought was 100%
the right thing in my mind,
was really the best thing
for me now.
But still somehow
I knew deep in my heart,
I made the right decision.

Now if only I could make it
through the fear along the way.
What if I'm wrong?
What if it doesn't work?
Who will be there for me
in my new life?
My anxiousness is overwhelming,
but I know this is what I need.

I smile on the way
through the doors
to the operating table,
And can't wait
to start my new life.

3/18/95

Σ

24. My Preop Experience

"Preop" refers to anything they do to you right before surgery. When we got to the hospital, a nurse checked me into my room. Since I did the pre-admitting part the day before, most of the paperwork was done. I remember being given a robe to put on and then medical personnel coming into the room putting intravenous lines into my arms, checking my vital signs, and giving me medication. Kay and I were talking a lot and trying to keep each other laughing. I didn't want any of my other family members to get there until after I was prepared because I knew it would only make them nervous and that wouldn't do anybody any good. I was used to taking tests and visiting the hospital, they weren't.

Don't get me wrong! I love my family very much, and they were very supportive at this point. But when I'm in a situation where my health is being affected, I need all the strength I can get. So for me, the fewer the people, the better I do. And I think they understood.

I think there are two different kinds of people in this world when it comes to being sick. There are the ones who want the whole world to know and there are the ones who just want to be left alone. The ones who want everyone to know will "milk" their relatives and friends and anyone who will listen to them to give them sympathy. The more the better is their attitude. They love the attention and feed on it. Needless to say, this group generally tries to avoid surgery. Surgery might make them well and then they'd have nothing to talk about.

The other extreme is the group of people who tells no one

when something goes wrong. This group sees any kind of sickness or health problem as a weakness. They fear it will control their lives in some way and don't want to take the chance that anyone will find out. It will make them vulnerable and others might try to take advantage of them under these circumstances. They see adversity as something that needs to be overcome, not something that you give in to.

Personally, I don't think it's healthy to be on either extreme. I will just say that writing this book has been my attempt at dealing with my past and trying to balance my views a little. If we could all fall somewhere in the middle of these two extremes, we'd probably turn out okay. So maybe we'd better get back to the good part.

Dr. Bruce came by to see me. He wanted to remind me to take it easy after surgery. "Hey kiddo, you are looking jolly good! Are you ready?" I just said, "More than ever! Are you ready?" He responded, "I'm always ready!" You know, I was sure that he was! Dr. Bruce has this confidence about him that says everything is in control! He is also Scottish, very charming, and has this unique way of expressing himself that kind of makes you want to listen to what he has to say. He continued, "I know this is going to be hard for you, but try to be patient. After surgery, you will feel very tired for quite awhile. Your energy will come back, but you have to be patient!" I responded, "Okay, when can I go jogging?" He chuckled, "Well, we'll see!"

I thought the surgery might slow me down, but I was in great shape, and I figured I'd be out of bed in a couple of days. I didn't need to rub it in anyone's face, though. I could show off after my operation, and everyone would be so impressed with my quick recovery.

About this time I think the "goofy juice" was beginning to take affect. This is the drink you are given that makes you feel really good just before you pass out. Kay and a couple of friends video-taped the whole thing, probably to hold me accountable for anything I said or did. Personally, I don't think this was quite fair, but I have to admit that I enjoyed it later.

Within about ten minutes, I sounded like I was drunk but kept telling everyone that the "juice" didn't work. Actually, I was scared that if they didn't give me enough medication to knock me out, I'd wake up during the surgery. So if I had any fear at this point, that was it!

What I didn't realize at the time was that the anesthesiologist takes care of the patient during surgery. I would be getting a lot more medication put into my body throughout the rest of the day. This juice drink was just the beginning.

My parents came by to see me, as well. I was really happy to see them, but also knew that I had to limit my communication time just before surgery. So I told them how much I loved them, and how happy I was to have this opportunity. I wanted to go into this operating room knowing that if something did go wrong, I'd be on really good terms with everyone and at peace with the most important people in my life. It was the perfect preop experience!

The last thing I remember was talking and laughing with people, exactly what I wanted before going into the OR. I remember telling everyone how silly it was for the hospital staff to think that a little fruit drink could knock me out. The next thing I remember wasn't so pleasant. One minute I was laughing and having fun, the next minute I was waking up in excruciating pain.

Σ

25. My Surgery Experience

Part I. ICU

I was waking up in the ICU and didn't know what was going on. I remember feeling really, really sick. My head was killing me, and I was very nauseated! I wasn't sure which was worse. I've never felt this bad all at one time in my whole life! Well, you want me to be honest, don't you? It is no fun waking up after a temporal lobectomy.

My whole body felt totally traumatized. I would describe it as being hit by an eighteen-wheeler. The only thing I knew was that it was going to take every bit of energy that I had just to get well...and I wasn't sure if I had that much.

Everything seemed so confusing and so overwhelming. I must have been falling in and out of sleep. Why did people keep waking me up and why did they keep turning on those bright lights that made my head hurt so bad? Why were people talking so loud? Why couldn't they talk to each other and not me? Better yet, why couldn't they just go away? Why won't they leave me alone? Why won't my head stop hurting?

It was like I was having all of these sensations at one time, and my brain wasn't able to process everything quick enough to keep up. I think maybe our brains have a difficult time sorting out the information and making sense of everything after the surgery. It's like our senses can't figure out how to process sound, light, taste, touch, and smell all at the same time without feeling overwhelmed. Any kind of processing takes a lot of concentration, and it all gets mixed up together. I want to really emphasize this because I think it will help people who want to help us. It's hard to understand the concept of your brain having to think to process things that are automatic for us normally, like our senses. Without saying it, I was thinking, "How do I make everything stop? I can't take in this much information all at one time! Help! I can't keep up! This is too hard! I don't understand! Make it stop! Just make everything stop!"

Part II. My Recovery

The next day, they moved me into my hospital room. I was starting to process information a little quicker. I felt like I could talk without getting too overwhelmed. It was hard, but I was moving forward at least.

Another way to explain it would be that your brain is trying to put the big picture together, but the pieces to the puzzle are all scattered about. And some of the pieces may not even be available. We have to find those pieces that are missing before we can begin.

On top of that, you will be in a lot of pain. The nice part is that the surgeon doesn't have to cut through a lot of muscle like on other parts of our bodies, so we don't have to worry about physical therapy. I thought I should throw in that positive message while I am telling you about all of the crappy stuff.

Dr. Bruce came by to see me as well. He has this way of making the room light up when he is in it. I felt so loved and so special whenever he was around, and I was always so happy to see him! It's kind of like all of your problems just disappear when you see him smile. Apparently, I was talking quite a bit and this was a good sign. I don't know, but I didn't feel like I was in as good of shape as he did. For some reason though, that didn't matter! I knew when I saw him smile, I could do anything!

By the second day, I had stopped taking morphine for the pain when I realized that it was doing me more harm than good. A part of the problem with this surgery is that you have to be under so much anesthetic and then after surgery, they want you back on your seizure medicine as well. When you have so much medication running through your system, you feel really sick. Unfortunately, there's not a lot we can do about it. But you don't have to take the morphine. You will definitely want something for pain, but try something milder if you can. The morphine just made me really nauseated mixed with all of that other stuff. It's really hard! But now that you have all of this wonderful information, it'll be a piece of cake for you, right? Just don't go out and run a mile the day after surgery, and make me look bad, okay?

By the second or third day, they gave me Zofran to help me feel better. I was having dry heaves and begging for something stronger. I found out later that Zofran is used for the prevention of chemotherapy-induced nausea and vomiting. No wonder it worked so well. They may not tell you about it at first because it's very expensive and not as readily available. If the regular stuff works for you, you won't need the Zofran.

Depending on the type of surgery you have, you may be out of the ICU within twenty-four hours also. The downside to this is that they want you out of bed and walking to the restroom to take care of business. I'll tell you, I did not want to get out of bed and walk to the bathroom no matter how bad I had to go. They could have just left that catheter in me, and then this wouldn't have been a problem.

When I first got out of bed, I was very unstable. I couldn't believe it. I was in such great shape, I thought. How could walking to the bathroom be that hard and that scary? I remember a nurse helping me the first time out of bed. I felt so weak, I hated it! It was like it took my mind a really long time to tell my body what to do. Isn't that weird? That experience was the next clue that it was going to take a long time to get my strength back.

There is something else you will need to know. It will take energy to talk. Don't get too worried because the words will come to you just like they did after the grand mals. Try not to think about it. I always found that whenever I started to get worried about it, I'd start stuttering, and I think it was more because I was nervous. If you can be around people you are comfortable with, you will heal much better and much faster.

If you feel like you absolutely have to keep your defenses up around certain individuals, try not to be around them. It will take energy for everything, and having to keep a wall up will be too much work. Just think of the surgery as having a very large grand mal seizure. Except this time when you recover, it's possible you may never have seizures again.

Σ

26. Brain Surgery:
The Rehabilitation Process

Your physicians will probably tell you to allow two months to start feeling like yourself again, and I won't argue with that. But I will say that it took me more like six months before I really felt like my confidence came back.

I was in the hospital five days before they asked me to leave. I'm sure this must sound funny, but I got used to being there. For me going into surgery was nothing compared to going home from the hospital. I was really scared to leave. I started crying every time I thought about it. I was so worried, but tried to hide it. I kept thinking about all of the terrible things that could happen after I left the hospital. Who was going to be there for me? How was I going to start over? What happens if something goes wrong with my brain after I leave the hospital? Who will know? What will I do? What will happen then?

I felt like I had so much to prepare for. Should I be preparing for the future or worrying about some post-surgical problem that won't be discovered until its too late? If you have any of these thoughts going through your head, I want to reassure you that I did too. So either you're not crazy, or both of us are crazy. I'll leave that up to your own judgment!

So leaving the hospital is going to feel weird, to say the least, and I think it's one of the scariest things you will do. All you can do now is to wait. You've already taken the biggest step there is by going through the surgery when all else failed. What you have now is time. All you can do now is wait, rehabilitate, and think positive. If you are a religious person, I'm sure it wouldn't hurt to say a few prayers.

I don't think physicians really understand this part of the rehabilitation process. Maybe their fear is before the surgery or getting us through surgery and back into the real world again. It's almost like they don't really understand why we still need them as we are getting well. They forget that they were the ones we've shared some of our biggest secrets with. My doctors knew everything about me. And they accepted me! Why would I want to leave them?

In the hospital I had very good treatment. I'd say I had five or six doctors checking on me while I was there. But the irony is that not one of them acted the least bit nervous about releasing me. I'm sure it was just that they wanted me to get back into the real world as soon as possible, and not that they were tired of me telling them what to do.

On the day I left the hospital, everything seemed so exaggerated. Normal sounds were louder than usual, people's voices sounded like noise, lights appeared really bright, and everything was moving so fast. I couldn't keep up. Okay, I have an example. Compare living in a small country town with very little action to your first experience visiting downtown New York City on a busy night. How's that for a comparison? That's what it felt like leaving the hospital. Here's what happened.

Kay did the honor of checking me out of Medical City and letting me stay at her place for the first week. I remember getting in her car and driving to her house. It was a nightmare! She drove a Nissan 300ZX. That didn't help matters. She always liked fast cars. I remember once when this young guy pulled up next to us in a new Mustang. Actually, we were going through a tollbooth and he started to rev-up his engine a little. Kay looked at me, and I said, "Go for it!" We did!

The next thing I remember was going around a turn and the other guy's car skidding out. I looked at her, and she said, "Well, he could have beaten me if his car could've taken that turn. My car is better on turns. Mustangs are better on straight-aways. We got him on that turn, alright! His car can't handle 130 miles per hour on a turn like mine can!"

Anyway going home from the hospital, she was being very good. I checked her speedometer just to be sure. She was only going 60-65 miles per hour, but on that day it felt more like 130. And just being outside in the light made my head hurt.

I sure hope you have some patient people in your life. If you don't, try to make friends with some right before surgery. They'll come in handy later on. I think Kay knew I was scared by the way I was acting. Normally fast was fun, but after brain surgery, just getting in a car felt like a huge risk.

By the second week I was back in my apartment. Kay and I were driving each other crazy and for the good of our relationship, it was time for me to go home.

To walk through my front door was a good feeling. You know that feeling after you come home from a vacation? Maybe I should specify, a bad vacation. The kind of vacation where you can't wait to get home? Well it was like that, except better!

This healing process is a weird time because you are counting every day that you don't have seizures. If you ever did a drug protocol, you'll remember writing down all of your seizures and times that you took medication. You will still need to keep track of the auras because your neurologist is going to want to know how you are progressing. But now, you will really be focused on how many days you can go without having a seizure. It's scary and fun at the same time.

I stopped keeping track of my seizures and medication about a year and a half after surgery. Somewhere along the way I didn't need to write it down any more. I think writing it down helped me to accept the idea that it was over. After living a certain way for so long, it's too dangerous to accept change too soon.

It also kind of doesn't feel real. I think the whole experience is very overwhelming to our brains and putting our thoughts on paper is like trying to understand everything. Writing down your feelings kind of validates the reality and makes it feel more real.

It also allows you to keep track of your thoughts so that you can put them into a book one day--if you so choose.

As I am putting this book together, you understand that I can only give you my perspective, and my perspective is based on the adjusting period to becoming seizure free. I think there is a certain amount of change that occurs in a person after living through a traumatic event, any kind of traumatic event. The point is that after that experience you will be changed in some way, forever. Hopefully, in a good way, but still you will be affected. How you learn to cope with your past has everything to do with your future. Your ability to adjust will be your permanent mark on life.

I'm not making a judgment call. I'm just saying that our ability to adjust determines where we end up, good or bad. I suppose that's why this book is so important to me. I don't know that I have adjusted too well. I had this great big idea of how the world was going to be and should be, and maybe I was a little disappointed. There was something about surviving that I enjoyed. When it was all over, I wasn't too sure what to do. Does that make sense, or does that make me a martyr?

My doctors told me that it would take awhile for me to adjust to being seizure free, but I didn't get it. I thought I'd have surgery, get well, and then do everything I was already doing but more of it and better, and it would be easier. Well, that's kind of true but not completely. I'll explain why in more detail in Chapter Thirty-One. But don't jump ahead, we still have lots of good stuff to talk about before we get there.

I was so anxious to get back to work that I called and told them I'd come back in after my third week postop. This was the longest I had ever gone without having a seizure, and I wanted to see how it was going to feel doing what I loved to do--working on people's hair. I wanted to start my life over right away. I didn't want to miss out on anything while my brain was still working.

Part of my problem was that I did not allow myself grieving time. I was so excited to be given a "new lease on life" as my therapist calls it, that I didn't want to think about the past or about the trauma of what I had just lived through. I wanted the good life back that I had before the seizures started, and I wanted that life to begin now, right now!

The first day I went back to work, I only lasted about three hours. I strongly recommend that you start back in increments, a few hours at a time is good. This will give your brain time to adjust and for you to build your stamina back. Even if your surgery is entirely different from mine, I'm quite sure that you will feel drained when you first start back to your normal routine. My hardest part was being patient. It felt like my energy was never going to come back.

So this first day at work, I didn't last long. I would go to the back room catch my breath between clients, and by the third hour, I was back there crying. A couple of the women I worked with cared enough about me to tell me to go home. They promised they'd call me if they needed anything. With that in mind I felt a little better, and I took off the rest of the day.

I constantly had this feeling of wanting to hurry up and do everything before it was too late. I even got anxious when people would call and ask how I was doing. I was afraid anything could jinx my luck so the only real hope I had was to pretend the seizures never happened in the first place.

When someone asked me if I was still okay, it reminded me that at one time I was not. I didn't want to know that because I couldn't afford to accept it. I felt like people were being rude by not going along with my denial. Why didn't they understand that I wanted to feel like I had this wonderful freedom that couldn't be taken away? I didn't want to be reminded that it might end again. I never wanted to hear the words, epilepsy or seizure, ever again!

My perspective was that I better hurry up and enjoy my free life, before it ends again. It had only been three weeks, but that was like a real successful adventure for me. Those were the most successful three weeks I had had in six years, and I wanted to celebrate in a very big way. The only thing I could think of doing was to go cut people's hair.

We had a good time at that salon. There's something about

a part time job that makes it so enjoyable. You get to show up long enough to have fun, but not long enough to get caught up in everybody's problems. It's kind of like the seriousness of everything is removed when you are a part-time employee. You also get to be the hero by coming to save the day when the shop gets really busy.

We used to laugh about everything, especially ourselves. We'd take turns talking about the silly stuff that happened during the week and how we were going to remedy the situations in our lives. We talked a lot about our relationships, as well. We'd discuss who was in the worst shape and then laugh about it. It always seemed like no matter what was going on in my own life back then, I could go to work and feel better about my problems.

As I became more well, my need for the salon would disappear. This is the part of my life that my brilliant doctors were trying to warn me about. In order to attain what I needed and wanted out of life, now, I would have to lose what I had always loved!

It's kind of like a part of you dies after surgery. That's the best way I know how to explain it. Things that brought me gratification were not bringing me much satisfaction any more. I think this is a very normal process in life but we don't notice it because normally it is so gradual. With surgery, it was like I had aged overnight. How I communicated with people, how I reacted to situations, how I lived my life, all of it would have to change if I were to be successful now.

How Much We Care

Isn't it funny how
much we hold inside.
How much we dream
and how little we care.

We walk around in a daze
and wonder why
life goes by
so hard and so fast.
Can we dream of yesterday?

What happens
to the memories
we want to keep
but can't find a way?
What we learn to say
we hear our own way.

The path leads us
to our dreams
if we follow our hearts,
And an open door
allows us to enter
to what we know is right.

Up the road
to a nice warm place
where we can
feel good inside.

Isn't it funny
how much we dream
when we can already
see the light?
How much we care!

6/3/95

Σ

27. Postop Depression

About two months after surgery, I started feeling really sad and wanted to cry a lot. Dr. Bruce says that "your brain misses the seizures." Maybe certain neurotransmitters are released or affected during seizures that make our brains feel good. Without the seizures, our brains miss those substances, and we become depressed. It's only speculation, of course, but why do mental hospitals give severely depressed patients electro-convulsive therapy? That's kind of funny, huh? Here we are removing the mechanism giving us seizures and making our lives hell. And at another hospital they are inducing seizures to make their patients feel better. Okay, I guess that's kind of serious, but you can see the humor in it, can't you?

In addition to this biochemical response from our brains missing the seizures, we also become depressed as a result of a major surgical trauma to our bodies. Maybe a good example of this would be how a woman becomes depressed about a month after delivering a baby. She's excited and happy with her new baby, however, her body is still adjusting to all the changes it must go through.

This is a difficult reaction to explain because we think we are supposed to be happy, but we are feeling sad. The best advice for me to offer is to be aware of these changes so that if you do start feeling depressed, you will know that your body and brain are just making adjustments.

Making adjustments and being depressed brings up another issue--grieving. To me, grieving always sounded like such a negative thing, like a continuous process of being sad that would never end. I don't think that is what is meant by grieving. I do believe that grieving can be a positive thing if it is a way to accept the bad things that happen to us, cry about those things and even allow ourselves to be depressed and angry, but then move on. I think the key here is moving on.

I wrote this poem in August of '95, about four months after surgery. I think it puts the seizure disorder into a perspective that you will be able to relate to.

A War

The closer the instability is
to your immediate environment,
the worse the stress as a result.

A War,
in another country, okay.
A War,
in your country, not okay.
A War,
in your city, really bad.
A War,
on your street, intolerable.
A War,
in your house, not livable.
A War,
in your head, then where?

[I didn't have an answer back then, now I do.]

A War,
in your head, complete imprisonment.

Σ

28. Post-Traumatic Stress

You've probably already heard of post-traumatic stress. Whenever we undergo any kind of traumatic event, there is a certain amount of denial that goes on in our minds while enduring the trauma. When we are far enough away from the danger of the situation, we will begin to come out of denial, along with accepting the severity of what we have just lived through. During this time, we may start feeling anxious and scared all over again.

For me this time came about two months after surgery. I think all of my post-traumatic stress came from living with seizures rather than from the brain surgery. The surgery was planned, and it was a one time event. I figure anyone can deal with one traumatic situation in life and still be okay.

Living with epilepsy was day in and day out. The seizures were never planned, and I never knew how bad they were going to be once they started. I didn't know who I could trust or who would try to use the seizure disorder against me once they found out. Epilepsy never ended! The stress never ended! The surgery was like a miracle cure. Okay, it was painful, and it was also hard to recover from. And yes, a lot changes afterward that we have to adjust to and to live with. But when you've lived with seizures and medication, surgery and recovery seems like a piece of cake by comparison.

Anyway, this post-traumatic stress may be something we have to live with for the rest of our lives. Not in a really bad way, but to some extent I still get scared. When I first started *Seizure*

Free, it was a way to deal with what happened to me. A couple of months after I had been working on the book, I had this nightmare that I was having a seizure in my sleep. I woke up sweating and couldn't get back to sleep so I lied in bed for awhile and told myself that it wasn't real. I finally fell back to sleep, and by morning I forgot about it, kind of. Okay so I told myself to remember so that I'd be sure to include that story in the book. It seemed like the right thing to do. Is that better?

This is going to sound a little weird, but you may experience some post-traumatic stress with seasonal change. As the weather changes, you will remember how you were feeling the previous year at that time. It is perfectly normal to start feeling scared all over again. But knowing this may happen might prevent you from undue stress.

I've got another thing to say about this "adjusting to being seizure free." I think they should call it, "trying to trust your brain again after all that it has put you through." The truth is that you never completely get back that feeling you had before the seizures started. My therapist tried to explain this to me.

I remember going to see Kathie after surgery. It was kind of fun sitting in that chair again where I had been sitting for the last two years trying to figure out why I was having seizures. Only now I was in a completely different place. I was rehabilitating, and I was on a different road. The problem had been solved! I don't mean solved because of the surgery. I mean because of the monitoring. They had found something wrong with my brain, and I could relax now. I could sit in her office without the fear that I did something wrong, without the fear that some deep-rooted issue was causing me to have seizures, and without the fear that I would discover this horrible secret that would end my life.

So I went back to see Kathie while I was adjusting to my new life, and I remember feeling a little sad one day. The tension was gone, most of the stress was gone, but something was still missing! So she asked me what the problem was, and I told her, "Something's missing, Kathie! I remember how I used to feel when I was twenty-four years old, before the seizures started, and I remember how I used to believe that anything was possible. I felt so in control of my life and so on top of the world. That hasn't come back, yet? How do I get that feeling back?" She just looked at me with amazement, leaned toward me, and tenderly explained, "Leanne, surgery may have cured the seizures, but you still had to live with epilepsy, and that experience will stay with you forever." I sure didn't like hearing that, but I knew she was right.

I was living in this world of "what if...what if this never happened? Let's pretend! Let's start over! Let's start back where we left off and let's see what happens!" I had this belief, without ever saying it, that I would get back something I lost. I would get back my perspective, not just my freedom.

I do know that it got better with time, but I also know now that I would not want that perspective back. That perspective came with its share of problems, and I certainly would like to believe that I've grown considerably since then.

Anything could have happened! It doesn't really matter what it was. Everyone will have something to overcome at some point in their lives that will change their perspective forever. The point is that we have to have hope, no matter what. We can't get our innocent lives back, but we can still have hope!

For about the first three years after surgery, I'd get this over-whelming feeling that something was going to destroy my life. I felt like I couldn't put too much importance on anything or something bad would happen to end it. I didn't care what was going to happen as much as I cared about being able to plan for it. When the seizures started, I didn't have any warning. It was like one day my life was great and I was making all of these plans, and the next day my life was ending.

I know that things happen to all of us or they wouldn't call it life. But I still felt like I should mention this fear that has lingered for quite some time, just in case you feel something similar. I'm 100% positive that it has to do with the seizures, but like I said before, maybe something else would have come along. And maybe that something else would have been worse. Who knows?

I know that I have it pretty good right now, and that I am

going to make the most of this situation that I possibly can. Tomorrow may be different, and I will deal with that when it comes. But today, I'm going to make a difference!

Σ

29. The First Six
Months Seizure Free

During the first six months after surgery, I couldn't believe
how good I felt. Everything was such a big deal but in a very good
way. I was doing everything that I did before but more of it. This
was a very special time for me. Every experience I had was a
monumental event. Every place I went, everything I did, every
person that I met, every feeling that I had, and every thought that
entered my head--all of it was very special! It's kind of like getting to be a kid all over again. Everything is new, innocent, and
fun!

You may be coming off medication from time to time. As I
recovered, I felt like the medication was becoming stronger. Maybe
my brain was no longer needing it, so the side effects were more
noticeable. About every two months I would get my meds reduced,
until one day I would no longer need them.

Reducing medication is scary because you don't know at
what point you will have a seizure and have to go back on more
medication. It feels like a test to see how well your brain is going
to function on its own. I want to stress that this is not a test we
have any control over. If you have a seizure at any point, it's okay.
It just means that maybe you will need to remain on your medication for a little while longer, or maybe always.

But you have come a very long way, and you are successful
just for surviving this. I'm saying that because of how I felt. I was
constantly worried that I was going to fail, and the problem is that

this seizure stuff is not a matter of failing. It's a matter of we want to be as well as we can, and we do everything to get there, but that's it. I know the seizures can still come back, but I could be hit by a drunk driver tomorrow, too. Some things we just don't have a whole lot of control over, so it's better to enjoy what we do have while we have it. I'm sure you get the point!

Coming off medication is so different from having to go on it. The normal procedure for me before surgery was to have seizures, increase my medication, get used to the side effects, have more seizures, increase the medication one more time, get used to the side effects again, have more seizures, and then start all over with a new medication. Does this sound familiar?

Well, I have good news for you! Coming off meds is almost exactly the reverse of what we are used to. Each time I felt too intoxicated, Dr. Leroy would decrease my medication level by a certain amount, and I'd get to feel good again. Cool, huh? I'd start feeling good, and the seizures wouldn't come back. This part was hard for me to believe. So then about a month and a half would go by, and I'd start feeling dizzy again. We'd just reduce my medication one more time. I'd get to feel good all over again, and I still wouldn't have any seizures. I know this is sounding too good to be true.

I really hope everything goes well for you if you do decide to have surgery because getting well is the neatest experience in the entire world. Maybe I should clarify that. If you've never had a seizure in your life, you probably wouldn't want to start having them so that you can live through years of medication and treatment that doesn't work too well, thinking it's all your fault, just so that you can experience this big procedure that involves removing a part of your brain so that you can experience the sensation of coming off of medication and becoming seizure free. But, for the rest of us, this is the coolest experience in the world! At this point I really don't think I'll find anything bigger, but I'll let you know if I do!

A Permanent Vacation

You ask me how I'm feeling
and I am free to say,
I'm on a permanent vacation,
a high that lasts throughout the day.
A 24 hour vacation from my fears
and relaxation without tears.

It's hard for me to believe
That I am still alive,
Today it occurred to me
That maybe I died.

I have gone to heaven
and maybe none of this is real.
But what about my family and friends,
why are they still here?

How could this have happened to me,
and how long will it last?
I'm a free person in a new environment,
should I forget about my past?

It's hard for me to believe
That I am still alive,
Today it occurred to me
That maybe I died.

I can go to sleep now
and know when I awake,
I will still remember today.
I will remember what I did,
what I studied, what I learned,
and what I said.
I will remember the people in my life.
Do you know how good it feels
to be on a permanent vacation?
Do you know how good it feels to be me?

SEIZURE FREE

Now, I can do anything
and become anything,
For I am free to travel where I choose.
I have a new lease on life
that few will ever receive.
Can you imagine what it feels like to be me?

It's hard for me to believe
That I am still alive,
Today it occurred to me
That maybe I died.

8/7/95

122

Σ

30. The Second Six Months
Seizure Free: Helping Others

I was getting a lot of confidence in a lot of different areas of life, but the best part was how much I was enjoying it. After the first month, my brain felt like it was on this wonderful vacation. I wasn't having seizures, and my thoughts were getting more organized. Just that one month vacation from seizures made a big difference. For every month that followed, I just felt like I kept getting smarter.

When I got to start reducing the medication, it got even better. Do you remember that show, "The Bionic Woman?" That's how I felt, seriously! I began to wonder what Dr. Bruce did to my brain. I'll tell you something else. I started thinking that maybe I was an experiment of some sort and they didn't want to tell me. Okay, I know this sounds a little crazy. But what would you think? You lived for what felt like an eternity with something that was destroying your life, you had just about given up hope, and then you get this great life with a brain that all of a sudden starts working really well, almost too well! It just doesn't feel real! And it doesn't make too much sense, either!

But I didn't care, I was going to enjoy every minute of it! During this time, I enjoyed helping other people in school. For the first time in my life I was explaining the material to other students, and that was in chemistry. To make it even better, I had never had a chemistry class ever in my life. Most of my youth I had been told that I had learning disabilities. It really bothered me a lot because Kay and my brother, Johnny, could get into the better schools, and I couldn't pass their tests. So I stayed in public schools until the sixth grade. The cool part is that I actually enjoyed my elementary school. So I guess there's a trade off to everything in life. Who knows, maybe I got the better deal?

I think a part of my problem in school is that I wasn't too good at sitting still. If I wanted to learn something, I'd go learn it. I didn't really understand why it was so important for someone to stand over me in the learning process. After surgery, though, I found a reason to be interested in school, and I did rather well!

Supposedly with this operation, your IQ can't change. But when you have a short-term memory that is functioning properly, your brain is not short-circuiting, and you are not intoxicated from medication, school sure becomes a lot easier. I know because I was on the Dean's list for the last year of college, the "good" Dean's list.

Under stress I still had trouble finding the words I needed to express my thoughts, but I was improving in areas of my life that I had never done well in before. I also think I know why. First, I began to have a huge interest in science, and I'd work really hard to understand it. Second, with the seizures, I had to learn certain ways to function in order to help my short-term memory work better. After surgery, I was doing everything that I trained myself to do in order to function with seizures, only now it seemed like a piece of cake compared to where I had been.

About this time, I noticed something else. As the weather changed, my head would hurt really bad. It got worse with cold, rainy, or windy weather. It kind of felt like someone had just opened my skull and put ice on my brain. How's that for an analogy? I've heard a few other people say this was a problem for them as well. Just make sure you have a warm hat and some earmuffs with you before you go out for the first time on a cold, rainy, and/or windy day. If it's really windy, take the earmuffs for sure.

Now let's get back to the good news. The day was November 19, 1995, and I would take my last dose of Lamictal. This was the final test to see how well my brain would do without that last little bit of medication that I was still on. When your medication is reduced it is done over a period of time and so gradually that by the time you take your last dose, there's probably not much in your blood stream anyway. Well, that's the way my doctor and I did it. I didn't want any surprises, so it was done very gradually over a period of seven months from my surgery date.

Around the beginning of December, I had to observe one of the University's gymnastics competitions and then write some kind of report on it. It was on this night that I realized I would probably never have to take medication again. When I got home, here is what I recorded in my journal.

It's over! The war is over!

Tonight at the gymnastics game, I realized the noise was getting too loud. I asked my instructor if I could leave but apparently I didn't say why. I did say, "Well, when you have a part of your brain removed noise kind of echoes." I think I made her feel bad but that wasn't the intent. At that point, she said, "Well, okay you can go." Of course I said, "No, I can take it."

Later , I told her that I would never use that as an excuse unless I thought I had to. She responded, "Leanne, you have to understand, if you asked to leave because you felt sick or had a headache, I'd say okay. But that's not what you did. You just said you wanted to leave for a little while." Well, I did have brain surgery not too long ago, and she could have just trusted my judgment. But I also wanted to be treated like everyone else, and that's exactly what she was doing.

So I'm glad she told me. I need to learn to ask to take care of myself, but I hate to admit that anything can get to me like that. I stayed until the meet ended at 11:30 pm. I did have to go outside for a quick cry when it got too noisy, but afterward, I was okay. Leaving the gym, I felt absolutely fantastic. I was walking to my car and thinking out loud, "I don't have to do anything any more! I don't have to take medication! I'm Free!"

I'm sure this story is not much of a revelation for you, but to me, it was a turning point in my life. This was the first night that I had stayed up past ten p.m. in about three years and not had to worry about waking up the next morning.

After I got home, I stayed up an extra hour studying for a physics final. The final was the next morning. This was the first time since I had been in college that I had an opportunity to stay awake and study. Not too many students see staying awake to study as much of a gift, but believe me, it is! This would not have been an option before surgery. Getting less than eight hours of sleep would have put my life in serious danger, and then trying to take a final the next morning would have been completely out of the question. I realized at that moment what this meant for me. I truly had a freedom that many people with seizures would never know, and that most everyone else has always taken for granted.

I WAS NOW A FREE PERSON!

Remember, I didn't want to ask for help because I didn't want to be seen as weak. If you ask for help, you are admitting that something is able to defeat you, right? Well, I'm not sure about that. But I do think it's okay to ask for help when you need it. In fact, I ask quite a bit now. There's a difference between asking for help and not trying. As long as you are trying, most people feel privileged to help you. I am seeing this now, but I'm in a completely different place, and life is a lot easier.

I think when you are fighting for your life, but still want people to respect you and to treat you like everyone else, asking for help is a very big deal. If you ask for help, they might think you want special treatment. If you ask for help, people might think you are asking because you have epilepsy and start treating you like you are sick, or God forbid, like you are disabled. Then they'll never leave you alone!

This is a very hard thing to get past because there's always this little voice in the back of your head saying, "You are not as good as everyone else because you can't make your brain work."

So now you have a major inferiority complex to get past while you are dealing with the side effects from the seizures and medication, and still trying to figure out why you have a psychological condition causing all of your problems.

Asking for help may have had nothing to do with the seizures or the medication, but in my mind there was always that fear. So for me, asking for help created a lot of stress and anxiety. I can tell you that other people are not thinking about your seizures twenty-four hours a day. That is a perspective that only we know. So when you ask for help, their response is not going to be a reaction to your seizure disorder--it's going to be a reaction to a person asking for help. And for the most part people like to help because it makes them feel good.

I really did not deal with having seizures very well. I wish I could give you more ways for coping but the truth is that I'm not very good at it. I just don't like focusing on problems for very long. I only think about a problem for a short period of time, long enough to come up with a solution. Then I focus on the solution only and pretend like the problem doesn't exist. I focus on getting to the other side and think about how good it's going to feel once I get there.

I really believe that there is always a way around every problem and every obstacle and every misfortune that comes into a person's life, and there's something exciting about figuring out how to get to the other side. There's something exciting about trying to take the most negative thing that exists and trying to turn it into something positive. I just focus on what I want until I get it, and then I try to deal with reality later.

The down side to being this way is that we are left with invisible scars that we eventually have to deal with. The upside is that we can recover quickly and feel accomplished in a very short period of time. We appear successful to the rest of the world even though we still have residue from our experiences that lingers for quite some time. That residue does gradually disappear over time, but not nearly as fast as we would like for it to!

Time to Reminisce

After all of this,
now the time has come
for me to reminisce.
It's still so overwhelming
to think that just last Xmas Eve
I didn't know where I'd be,
when today seems so easy and stress free.

I remember thinking
if I could have only one week
to do whatever I wanted,
or even one day
not to have to worry about survival,
surely, I'd be more thankful
for all that I have.

And I remember dreaming
of letting go of the fear
and thanking God for all that I had,
but instead of doing so,
I would just pretend
that it wasn't real
and I wasn't here.

Now I wonder what life will give me,
and if I will accept it.

11/19/95

Σ

31. The Second Year
Seizure Free: Why Me?

This was not a good time for me. I could no longer enjoy my new life without finding some reason or answer for having to have lived with epilepsy. I no longer felt the joy of getting to have my life back because the resentment of losing it in the first place was now taking over. I could no longer be happy because anger was setting in.

I'm supposed to be going on with my life, but what am I supposed to be doing? I can't go back to the person I was before the seizures started because I'm not really the same person. My perspective has been changed so much that the things that used to bring me joy are no longer rewarding. And I don't really have anything to prove any more, so why am I here?

The career that I wanted in my early twenties would seem meaningless and unfulfilling at this point. I loved doing hair and being self-employed, but going back in time didn't feel right either. Nothing felt right, and I didn't know what I was supposed to do about it.

I originally went back to school so that I could get a professional job and so that I wouldn't have to be self-employed the rest of my life. I thought if I could get a job in the field of kinesiology somewhere, then I could also get medical insurance. I was thinking that it would be a good idea to work with a large company that offered a lot of benefits, especially since I was getting older and I was having a lot of medical problems. The idea of a "benefits package" was sounding awfully good at that point in my life.

Being self-employed as a hairdresser, there was no such thing. When you have seizures, you take a cab to work. There was no such thing as sick leave, either. You found a way to pay your rent or you lost your lease. It was that simple!

It's really important to understand that just because we have brain surgery and get well, that doesn't mean our pasts have been removed. We still have to look at where we have come from to understand why so much changes.

It's like a good portion of your life has revolved around what you should and shouldn't do because of the seizure situation. Even if you are like me and went on with your life with epilepsy and tried not to talk about the seizures, your goals upon becoming seizure free, more than likely, will be a lot different.

Not having seizures changed a lot of things that I couldn't foresee changing, like certain aspects of my life. For instance, I realize now a good portion of what made school so interesting with seizures was the adrenaline I was living on. I hate to admit this, but when the adrenaline was removed, school became boring. I wasn't at all ready for this aspect of my life to be changed.

When you are having seizures there is a lot of risk involved in life. I suppose whatever I did, it would have been interesting because there's so much risk involved in living, that just getting through the day was a challenge in and of itself.

So this second year seizure free brought up a lot of issues. By this time I had forgotten why I was in school. I certainly didn't want to quit, but part of the reason I went back in the first place had been removed. I wasn't having seizures, and I wasn't on medication. Did I still want to work for someone else, and did I still need that degree?

I needed an answer and no one could give me one. It was like I was in this world that I didn't belong in any more, but I wasn't sure how to get out of it or how to get home. What I mean by home is how to get that feeling back, the gratification that I had gotten out of life, before I had surgery.

I also felt guilty about being depressed. I can say that now because it is quite obvious to me what the problem was. I was depressed and didn't know how to get 'undepressed.' My perspective had been changed and I didn't like that. Why couldn't I just get well and get gratification from the same things that I was getting gratification from before. Why did life have to become so complicated all of a sudden? Why did the good parts of my life have to change also? Even decisions had become harder to make. Decisions were always easy for me before, and now I couldn't make a decision to save my life!

It was easy to decide which way to go when I was having seizures because everything had to revolve around my health. You make the decision that will save your life. You decide and you don't look back!

When you are well, you have to take a lot of other things into consideration before calling life's shots. It's like your thinking becomes more revolved around other people and how your actions may affect those other people. You couldn't afford to think of these things before because you had no choice. Now you do!

So how I made decisions was changing, but so was my perspective of my environment. People who seemed so important and so impressive to me were no longer as successful as I had imagined them to be. It wasn't their fault my perspective had changed, but I was kind of angry that I didn't have these people to look up to any more. When I was having seizures, my goals couldn't possibly have exceeded theirs so they were very supportive. I was imagining doing their jobs in my condition, and that seemed very remarkable. And it would have been. Some of these "accomplished" people had now become some of the weakest people I knew. It wasn't anyone's fault, but I didn't want to know that! Maybe I was angry at myself, too! How could I have been so mislead?

You know that feeling you get when you go back to your hometown and see people that you used to look up to as a child? Well, you know that feeling when you realize these people are not anywhere near as successful as you pictured them to be, or as they may have wanted you to picture them to be? I think we've all had this experience at some point in our lives. I also think it's important to understand that if you feel this after you become seizure free, it is perfectly normal. Don't be mad at yourself for needing them at one time. It wasn't your fault!

Something else may happen after surgery that involves your interaction with other people. You may run into individuals who want to pity you. I see this behavior as sickening to say the least. I'm not talking about the people who are genuinely interested in your well-being. You can tell the difference. I'm talking about the ones who always need to feel sorry for somebody to validate the cruelty in the world and to justify their own shortcomings. This group will want to magnify your experience and then try to convince you that the world really is a terrible place because of what you lived through. If you don't mind my saying, let these people go. You are trying to heal, and you don't need any negative reinforcement while doing so.

Okay, I'll get off my soapbox. But can I say one more thing? I know that I did get that "pity" thing from some people, and it was humiliating to say the least. I felt like the people who wanted to pity me were not as successful as I was so I should be feeling sorry for them. The catch twenty-two is that I couldn't feel sorry for them because I secretly resented the hell out of them for having few obstacles to cross and doing little with what they were given. I also knew that I needed to hurry up and figure out what I was supposed to be doing with my life before I became one of these people needing to pity others to justify my own shortcomings.

So during this time since I was still in school and didn't know where else to go, I thought maybe physical therapy would be a neat occupation. I enjoyed learning about athletic injuries and for once in my life I was doing well in science courses. Actually, I was studying my butt off to do well in these classes, but they were so interesting that I wanted to learn more. There was also a challenge there that I didn't quite find in the other classes. Maybe that challenge could bring back the gratification that I used to get by being in school.

After my third day of observation at a physical therapy clinic,

I decided this was not going to be a good idea. Physical therapists don't get to diagnose. Since I was used to doing all of the diagnosing with my clients' hair, I kind of felt like I'd be ripped-off by someone handing me a prescription with the problem already solved. That kind of takes the fun out of it. The physical therapist has to decide what kind of equipment to use to help the injury and then has to take a bunch of notes afterwards. This didn't seem very gratifying at all, and I was pretty sure that you couldn't pay me enough to follow someone else's prescription.

It was toward the end of this year that I had become really depressed. I had already taken a bunch of the science classes as physical therapy prerequisites. But I was sure that I would hate it! What I wanted to do was to diagnose my patients' problems and to follow up with them to determine what the next step would be in their treatment. This meant that there was only one option left if I was going to work with patients. I had to become a doctor. My grades had been getting increasingly better since surgery, and I was doing relatively well in chemistry and physics.

That's it! I had epilepsy, I thought it was going to kill me for sure, and surgery saved my life. That had to be it--I was supposed to be a doctor. That's why this whole thing happened! God knew I'd survive and that I had a big mouth. I could become a doctor and help other people through their traumatic life experiences. This would put meaning to my entire life. These are the people who have done the most for me. They are the least selfish people in my life, they work harder than anyone else I know, and they are always the ones to encourage me to do more. That's it, I'm supposed to be a doctor!

Well, that's what I was thinking! But I also thought that all people who acquired some kind of illness would be obsessing to get well, like I was. I thought that all people loved their work and were embarrassed to have to call in sick. I thought that most people wanted to do more but were just being held back by something that is destroying their lives.

I'll tell you what happened. I was doing a cardiac rehabilitation internship as part of my kinesiology degree. Most rehab centers are set up in hospitals or near hospitals. They are established to help patients get back into shape after a heart attack or heart surgery. Interns will monitor blood pressure, fill out patients charts, and sometimes get to help with exercise prescriptions.

Anyway, I was doing this internship and thinking how lucky I was to be on the other side. For the first time I could see how it felt not to be the patient when I went to the hospital. What a deal! Unfortunately, it wasn't exactly a great deal. The patients weren't reacting the way I had expected them to, and I wasn't used to taking care of more than two or three people at a time. With hairdressing I could cut a client's hair while a perm was processing or style someone's hair while someone else was under the dryer, but I always had everything timed and organized so that I could stay on schedule and so that I could give each of my client's my complete attention. Everything felt important, and I could keep everybody happy!

This internship was not at all organized compared to what I was used to. I was supposed to take care of ten people all at once. Everyone is talking at the same time, no one is listening to anyone else, and I felt like I was accomplishing nothing. When I got to sit and listen to the patients and have some quality time with them, I'd go home feeling really good. But on the days that we had to rush through everything, I wasn't too sure that taking care of people was going to be all that rewarding. If I couldn't have quality time, I'd rather have no time! Also the science classes were becoming more difficult, and I was needing more time to study.

There was another very big problem with this internship. I didn't feel like I could tell anyone about my past because of the consequences if they found out. I'm supposed to be taking care of them so I have to keep my mouth shut and try to validate their feelings, right? They are supposed to be able to lean on me, and I should be able to allow them to do that.

If I were to say anything about my surgery, I would have fallen apart. And if the hospital had found out about the seizures or the surgery, they might have treated me like I was weak, stupid, or crazy. These were usually the responses that I got so I learned to keep my mouth shut. I didn't need anyone patronizing me, and I couldn't allow any negative criticism to enter my mind because I was still so fragile myself.

I'll tell you what happened, and I'm putting this story in here for those of you who have survived something that has changed you in some way and as a result left you resentful to others who did not have to go through your experience. During the internship, I was exposed to a few very ungrateful beings. There were also some people I really enjoyed, but unfortunately they didn't make up for the rest. Here's the scenario. A fifty-five year old woman who is seventy pounds overweight comes into the hospital after having a heart attack and I'm supposed to take care of her for the next few months. No problem, right?

I felt terrible for her.....until she opened her mouth. Every-day it was the same thing. Everything was someone else's fault. She complained constantly and wouldn't take any responsibility for anything. After two months of this, I was about running out of patience. I don't want to sound mean, but there was this little voice inside my head that wanted to say, "Lady, you have no idea how lucky you are! All you have to do is to lose weight and most of your health problems will be solved. I have lived six years of my life with seizures! I'm half your age, and I can't get those years back! All you've had is a little warning from God to take better care of yourself. Surgery for us (people with epilepsy) is a luxury, not a place they send us because we were too lazy to take care of ourselves. Now get over it! And be a little more grateful that you are on this planet and all you've lost is a couple hours of time in this hospital."

I guess it's pretty funny now, but I was so frustrated at the time. And I did eventually lose my temper on this one particular day. It was one of the noisiest days ever, and her negativity was not helping matters. I started out being really nice. I asked her if she would mind being quiet for a couple of seconds so that I could finish taking her blood pressure. I kept trying to be nice, but I was having a hard time holding back my true feelings. She just kept getting louder and louder, and more and more negative. And as

135

she did so, I could feel my own anger coming back. I could feel it coming out, and I couldn't hold it back! Okay, that's no excuse. There is never an excuse to lose one's temper. But I did! I finally said, "How am I supposed to do this with all of this noise in here?"

Well, she went and told my supervisor as if I had just told her she was the worst person on the planet or something. That was her excuse for not coming back, anyway. I'll tell you what. I had no right to get upset, but she was definitely looking for a way out. And I was it! This way she didn't have to accept the situation she had placed herself in, and she also wouldn't have to do anything about it. I suppose I don't blame her, though, I wouldn't have wanted to either.

The point is that my resentment allowed me no leeway in dealing with this conflict of interest. I feel really stupid now that I even allowed that situation to take place. I didn't understand that my feelings would eventually surface, and I didn't know that I'd have resentment for people who weren't more grateful for what they had. So much resentment, in fact, that I wouldn't be able to just smile and go on my way and ignore them. In my supervisor's office, I broke down and started crying. I was mad, sad, and confused. Why couldn't other people be more grateful? And why did I have to work so hard to get caught up? I just didn't get it! I didn't get it at all!

There is a lot of psychology to healing from brain surgery, and looking back maybe I should have just given more people a chance to come into my life. Maybe I should have been more open and I would have been able to get through the internship without losing my temper.

It's always easier to look back and say, "I should have....." But sometimes that's not possible. Today I can say a lot of stuff. This is my second edition of *Seizure Free,* and I'm feeling very comfortable with my position in life right now. I don't feel like a lot can hurt me so I can afford to be more open. At that time it may not have been a good idea. I did what I felt was necessary for the place I was in and for the people I was around.

So I was needing grieving time in a very big way, but I sure didn't want to take it. Couldn't I just pretend that I had a new life now and the old one didn't exist? Couldn't I just hurry up and do some kind of great thing and forget about the past? Absolutely not! Our pasts will always come back to haunt us if we try to run away, as I found out during the internship.

I really had a hard time justifying my feelings. That's funny to me now. I don't know anyone who can get through major brain surgery to fix a major problem that they have been living with for several years and then go back to work and pretend like none of it ever happened.

Some new responsibilities were about to enter my life, as well. Two months after surgery, I inherited a ranch with my brother and sister. I knew it might be difficult for all of us to agree with how to handle this situation, but I had no idea how many problems it would cause. With this new responsibility came new stresses that I wasn't at all ready to take on.

We knew that we didn't want to just have to pay the taxes on it, so the ranch would need to generate some income to pay its bills. We decided to continue to lease parts of the ranch for cattle, and to also set up hunting leases with some people that my brother knew. Although we had some routine family disagreements, it seemed like new opportunities were coming our way, and we were doing quite well financially. As a hairdresser, although I loved it, I never made that much money and it was a lot of hard work. This new ranch partnership was allowing me to go to school full-time and still pay the bills.

The point I'm making is that it was very hard for me to justify being depressed because I had so much, I thought! My brain was working, I was making money, and I should have been happy! Maybe! I didn't realize that I would need to find a way to fit into this new world that I had entered. My communication skills with people would have to change. Some of my interactions with people were no longer appropriate, and how I did business would have to be completely reorganized overnight if I were to be successful in this new life. I would need to grow up now. And I would have to do so very quickly.

Every aspect of my life had changed, and I would need to find new ways of getting gratification. The old ways no longer worked. They worked when I was having seizures, and they worked when I felt like my options were limited. But I was no longer in that place. I would have to rehabilitate from brain surgery and cross my fingers that the seizures didn't come back, but I would also have to learn new ways of communicating with people now that I was in a different place. I would have to say goodbye to the old life if I wanted to welcome the new one.

Here's the catch twenty-two. How much do you let go of when the seizures can come back tomorrow? How much responsibility should you push yourself into, when you know that you have no control, or I should say limited control, over the outcome of this surgery? This is a very big question, and it makes life confusing and difficult during the first couple of years after surgery. I want to make sure I validate this for you because it may clear up some problems.

Knowing this can be an issue allows us to understand the anxiety and the depression, but knowing how to handle it can be another issue. I wish I had gone on medication during this time because I think it would have helped me to deal with certain situations a lot better, and maybe I wouldn't have gotten caught up in some of the problems that I did. Until now, I've always been one to believe that a person should be strong. We should deal with our stuff and move on. That has always been my philosophy, and I think I've done a fairly good job at following it. However, I now believe that taking medication to help us move on is also okay and some times necessary.

If you are caught in this dilemma, your neurologist should be able to help you out. I know that now a lot of patients do go on antidepressants after brain surgery, but if you feel okay, you may not need to. I just wanted to add that because I think my life may have been a little easier to adjust to with medication.

It was like I had so many things in my life change after surgery that I was a little overwhelmed. My personal life was being reorganized for various reasons, and all of my goals and dreams were changing as a result of so much opportunity all at one time. When you are feeling good, it's okay to be overwhelmed. When you are depressed, it can do a number on you. I had a lot of feelings going on and a lot to try to sort out. On top of that, there's the fear of how long is this going to last? Can I afford to trust my brain after all that has happened? Should I be planning for the future? And if so, how far in the future?

I will say something good about this time. My follow-up appointments were quite rewarding. My physicians were always there to encourage me when I was in doubt. And I needed that in a very big way! I remember one of my follow-up appointments with Dr. Bruce. I was so excited that I was doing well in school and in science, in particular. I was trying to make all "A's" in my classes since my brain was working so well. When I told him that I got a "B" in physics, here is what he had to say about it. "You know, physics is where we lost most of our medical students. They just couldn't get through that part!" He always knew exactly what to say! So of course I went back to school with a big head and ready to take on the world!

When we get well, it's like a part of our lives have been removed and some of the people who were there for us, our doctors, have also been removed. It's like we go through this war with these people, and neither one of us has much of a choice about it. When it's over, it's over! But we also have to leave them behind. These people have seen us at our worst, and now we'd kind of like to make up for lost time. But we're supposed to just go on with our lives and forget about them, forget about the war, and forget about that life! That's hard to do! We want them to come with us and to enjoy the good stuff with us, too! They understand us and understand our problems. But we have to learn how to go on without them and without their support, and it's hard!

Where Do I Go From Here?

Where do I go from here
when I lost my sense of direction?
What I believed was my survival
has left my soul without possession.

It's a feeling of disbelief
that overcomes my well-being,
and not even this bit of grief
will relieve what I'm seeing.

A life full of promise,
youth, and goodwill
had too many offers
for success to fulfill.

I still wonder why
this new life makes me question,
just how much are we given
when so much has been taken?

And where do I go from here
with a new sense of direction?
Can I believe in this revival?
Will my soul find a new connection?

Maybe this isn't about time
or how much change one can survive,
but rather, an understanding
for what we learn,
and what we get out of life.

5/8/96

Σ

32. Two and a Half Years
Seizure Free: I Think It's Over

Here are some notes from my journal. I thought it would be better for me to include my actual feelings at the time instead of trying to recap everything now. This will give you a better idea of what I was feeling at exactly that time.

I had a deja vu today, earlier. I didn't have a seizure but tonight I went out. I was going to go by the bookstore but decided to drive by Parkland Hospital, instead. I remembered leaving the hospital in '93, after hearing that my seizures were psychosomatic and I could go home because there was nothing more they could do for me.

So why did I hold on for two more years? What enabled me to say, "I refuse to accept this!" I didn't want it to be a big deal, but now it is because I see now that nothing has meaning for me any more.

At least back then, I got so much meaning from everything in life. Everything was so important to me. Everyday mattered. And everyday made a difference. I lived for every minute because I never knew from day to day or hour to hour or minute to minute where I'd be. I had a reason to enjoy now. I had a reason to make the most of what I had because I didn't feel like I had very much.

*Today is different. I can't enjoy now
because I should be planning for the next twenty years.
I feel guilty if I enjoy today because I should be plan-
ning for tomorrow. And tomorrow doesn't matter either, it's just getting through whatever I have to go
through to attain the goal at the end of the twenty-
year plan.*

*Nothing is bigger than surviving a seizure dis-
order and brain surgery, so there must be something
waiting for me somewhere. God, I want to enjoy life
again!*

*I think most people are very spoiled. I don't
want to become like everyone else. I think I fit in more
when I had epilepsy than I do now.*

*A lot of the people that I worked with were
very poor. They were working to put food on their ta-
bles for their families, and I was working to save
money for brain surgery. They were not given the
luxury of a good education growing up, I was. Even
though we came from different backgrounds, we had
something in common--we were surviving!*

*Now, however, it's different. I don't understand
why they don't want to be educated, and yet, I don't fit
in with the people in college.*

*Before, I didn't have money or my health. Now
I have both! So where do I go? I can't go back in time,
but I don't know where forward is. Basically, I feel
like a total outcast.*

*I have a couple of friends that I can talk to,
but not so much about the past. I just try to lock it up*

and forget about it, and then hope some day that I really will.

So my only real goal now is to be happy. I don't think I'll ever get that feeling back that I had before the seizures started, but that may just be something that comes with age. When you're young, the world revolves around you and nothing bad will ever happen to you so long as you're a good person. Well, not so! And I suppose that not all young people are that naive. I was!

Something did come from this. I am much more sensitive to vulnerable people--not the ones who want you to feel sorry for them, but the ones who really are trying to make a difference in the world, only some obstacle is slowing them down. The truth is these people are few and far between. Most of us don't want to work. Most of us want to be given everything because it's easier that way.

I'm not sure how I feel about this. I never wanted anything to be given to me because I always felt like feeling good about what I had, was knowing that I had earned it. But the older I get, the more I "need."

Well, I am feeling much better now. Most of the sadness is leaving me. You know, next time I'm feeling lonely or sad or whatever, I'm going to write. Writing makes a difference for me. And maybe some day, it will make a difference for someone else.

July 21, 1997

Something I Lost

Part I. So far I've come,
down this road alone.
I'm looking back on my life
and wondering how to get home.

In this hierarchy of life,
it's a world of pretense.
So many to fight,
so few in your defense.

Who answers your prayers
when you're on your own?
In a world of transition,
so far from what you know.

I'm here by myself
wondering how I fit in,
why I have these opportunities,
and where I go to begin.

The Glory of Survival
somehow gives you a new outlook.
A chance to live your life over
and time to reflect on what it took.

3/1/97

Part II. Eight months ago
when I wrote those words,
I was grieving
for something I lost.

I now know where I've been
and just how much I've gained,
And I can tell you--
It was well worth the cost!

10/30/97

*I went to a women's poetry reading last night
and had a deja vu while I was there. Of course it didn't
turn into a seizure, but it made me remember how I
used to feel and the thoughts that went through my
head when I was in a situation with people around
me and I did have a seizure.*

*I better remind myself, it's been two years and
three months. I didn't have a seizure! That's no longer
a part of my life!*

July 27, 1997

I don't even remember what happened at that poetry reading because I was too busy trying to pretend that my past didn't
exist. Now I wish I had at least written some kind of funny story
for you.

All I can say is that you may still have auras for awhile.
Most of the neurologists and surgeons that I've talked to say that
the auras can continue for a couple of months after surgery, but
they may never turn into seizures.

For whatever reason, I had an aura on that night. I guess it's
just a feeling that used to precede the seizures so it kind of caught
me off guard. I'd say it happens about every three of four months
now but lasts only two or three seconds. I'm always a little concerned when I do feel it. I think it is something that someone
without seizures would call a deja vu. And it would be a normal
feeling for anyone else. But for us, it's a reminder of where we
came from.

This Trap

How did I manage to fall
into this trap,
when I spun the web
to weave in and out of the holes.
How did the last
tangled string
from my grasp?
Where did I miss the connection,
why didn't it last?

The answer was in front of me
all along the way.
The passion was the power
driving fear,
from here,
out of me.
Pushing out my feelings
to believe in life again.
Craving the freedom
I long to taste,
within.

So the spell has been broken,
and the power is released.
From within I taste a passion
burning to be free.
This spirit has a new motive,
a desire not driven by fear.
From here, I believe,
Control is not the answer.
From here, I believe,
I will be free.

8/6/97

Kay is in town visiting. She moved about a year ago out to California to fulfill her life long dream of becoming an actress. She told me that being in acting is about having a voice. If people recognize her, they will listen to what she says. She told me if she was a recognized actress, people would think she was important and then she could promote women's rights or anything else she believed in. She could make a difference because people would listen to her.

Anyway, she was supposed to be coming over for lunch. She called to say that she was going to be late, and here's how she opened: "Leanne, you know that feeling you get when you oversleep past your alarm, and you feel like you missed out on something and you want to go back, only you can't because now it's too late?"

Yeah, I knew exactly that feeling. There is a part of you that stays just a little sad when you think about your past. You can't go back and change it, and you can't pretend like you had a different one so that you'll feel better about who you are now.

When people ask what you were doing at certain times in your life, it's very difficult to explain why you were living a certain way without telling them your life story. Most people don't want to hear that you had brain surgery anyway, so it's usually just easier to avoid social settings that will force you into accepting their disapproval of you. I guess it makes me mad because this isn't what I wanted for my life story.

December 2,1997

I never used the seizures as an excuse but they made my life impossible. I noticed some time after surgery, I would get depressed when asked questions about my health. The problem was that I didn't have answers to simple questions because the last seven and a half years of my life had revolved around seizures, side effects from medication, taking tests for brain surgery, using experimental drugs for seizure control, and then rehabilitating from brain surgery.

I didn't know if I had allergies. I didn't know if I had PMS. I didn't know what my flu symptoms were. And I didn't know where too many places were because I had to give up driving.

If I had fever, I was sick. That was enough! If I had to get somewhere farther than two miles away, I found a ride, took a cab, or walked. If I had a headache, it was because of the medication or the seizures.

If I was depressed or angry, it was because we were trying a new medication and it took awhile to get adjusted in my system. For those of you who don't know, during this time we are more intoxicated than normal because we have to go off the old medication gradually while we are beginning the new one. This usually takes about two months or so.

I don't remember these inquiries bothering me before. They probably just made me feel more accepted. But after surgery, it hit me really hard. I remember Kathie telling me that this was a kind of "coming out of denial" that I was going through. I just felt like all of a sudden everything that anyone would ask me made me realize that the seizures had forced me to change more than I was accepting.

I didn't want to run away from people but I also didn't like feeling forced into accepting that my life revolved around a seizure disorder. It made me sad and mad all over again, and I didn't want to feel either one of these things.

I couldn't answer simple health questions because my life revolved around a much more serious issue, and I was now having to face this fact. How do you say to someone, "Pardon me while I start crying uncontrollably because it has just occurred to me that you and I have come from entirely different worlds." The problem is that you can't be mad at them for putting reality in front of your face. But how do you hide your pain to keep from looking stupid?

Looking back on this I can see that I was really not dealing with this change very well. Maybe I had lived in denial for so long that it was just really hard to accept afterwards. I also think that I was depressed and needed to be on medication. It's hard to know that when you are there.

It was like all of this trauma afterwards just wouldn't go away. I couldn't make it stop, I couldn't make it go away, and I didn't know how to accept it. No matter what I did, it was there reminding me how a part of my life was gone. Reminding me that I would have to start over, and reminding me that I was behind.

My Destination

I've grown apart
from this dream I call reality.
It's an opportunity
to take me back to the present
to proceed on this journey
we call life.

A time for a new beginning,
where a fragment of a second
could destroy the aspiration.
A chance to win
A chance to play
And time to change direction.

Walking on the line,
I could miss the revelation.
With a place to dream
and a place to feel,
the journey becomes my life.
And fate,
my destination.

11/27/97

Σ

33. So What Was Wrong with My Brain?

According to Dr. Bruce, the pathology lab found a drop of neurons in my sommer sector. Basically, that means I had scar tissue in my brain, the part they removed. It was probably from or at least partially a result of a rafting accident when I hit my head on a rock. I never went to a physician for treatment afterward because I didn't think that I had to. First, I was young and nothing could hurt me, and second, I was trying to get by on a very strict budget.

But I remember the accident quite well. I was with some friends, tubing down the Guadalupe River. As far as we knew, it was safe. Everyone tubes down the Guadalupe at some point in their lives if they live in Texas. It wasn't supposed to be that dangerous! We were just having fun like everyone else.

The next thing I remember was getting pulled away from the group by a current. The water was running quickly. At this point, I wasn't too concerned because I was a fairly good swimmer. As a kid at summer camp, I had to swim a mile and I was one of the first ones to finish. I loved water!

Anyway, the current began to pick up its speed and somehow I got pulled under. Before I knew it, I was getting pulled deeper and deeper, and I wasn't strong enough to fight the current. The next thing I knew my head had hit a rock somewhere along the bottom. I remember telling myself to just swim to the surface and to worry about it later, but for some reason the water was fighting me. My head was fine, but I couldn't reach the top. I was struggling and beginning to wonder how much longer I could hold my breath.

I kept pulling myself up but it felt like every stroke I took was not enough to get my head above the water. I just kept pulling myself through the current trying to find a way out. As I reached the surface, I was gasping for air. I could finally breath again, and now all I had to worry about was getting home.

Some people in a raft saw me and gave me a ride down. I don't know if they were in any better shape than I was. They were drinking beer, and it was quite apparent they had been drinking for some time that day. They were quite perplexed as to why a young woman by herself was struggling to swim down the Guadalupe without any protection.

To this day I'm not sure if they ever got the whole picture, but I didn't care. People being rescued can't be picky! The way I saw it, I had a better chance of survival with a bunch of drunks on a raft than I did alone in that cold water with the currents acting up. They were very nice. They offered me a beer and told jokes for the rest of the ride. I passed on the beer. I decided if I could focus on their humor, I could remove myself from the seriousness of the situation and forget about the fact that my head was bleeding, my heart was pounding, and my body was shaking. For some reason, I just couldn't get rid of the chills.

Well, we made it down the river although I'm not quite sure how. Isn't that the fun of life in our twenties? We do lots of crazy things, even things that we don't know are going to be crazy, and somehow we survive them all.

I think I was probably in shock after that little adventure, but I just figured that that was one of those unfortunate accidents that happens, and I should get over it. My head wasn't bleeding that badly, and it never occurred to me that I would need to follow up with a physician. I survived the river, so it was over! I just looked at it this way--I wasn't going to be doing any more tubing down the Guadalupe for awhile.

That may have been the beginning to the onset of a life with epilepsy, or maybe it was just one more thing to aggravate an already fragile neurotransmitting device that perhaps I was born with. I never recorded when we went to the Guadalupe so I will never know for sure if that was the point at which the seizures started or not. I do know that after my first grand mal seizure in my sleep, my neurologist at that time had told me that the deja vu feelings I had been having were really complex partial seizures. I was working about sixty hours a week trying to build my clientele and do hair shows with Redken. I just thought maybe I was having dizzy spells because I wasn't getting enough sleep.

I had febrile seizures as a baby but those disappeared in my childhood. Dr. Bruce says there is a higher incidence of adult onset of seizures in people who've had febrile seizures as infants, and with a head injury there is always a chance of aggravation to the brain.

With these things in mind, I was definitely in a higher risk category, but with no one in our family having epilepsy it was kind of a surprise. I will also admit that I did some recreational drugs in my youth, but that was dated. How could something so long ago out of nowhere make my brain do weird things? And why weren't those people who were with me also having seizures now? That part didn't add up, but with the other stuff against me, who knows?

The point is that it happened for what ever reason, and now it is over for whatever reason. This experience has left a major impact on my life in every way, and I have chosen to do something about it.

So why didn't the seizures show up on the EEG video monitoring in '93 the first time we tried to find the problem? The answer to this may be the best information I can give you. If your seizures are not big enough when doing the monitoring, your doctors may not be able to detect any abnormal brain wave activity. That doesn't mean it's your fault or that you are crazy, yet! Also, there is the chance that your seizures are coming from a deeper area in your brain and may never show up on an EEG. Again, you are not crazy, yet! I say that facetiously because of the jokes that go around in the EEG units. Dr. Leroy likes to joke with some of his patients, I assume it wasn't just me. When I'd go to see him on follow-up appointments, feeling really good that the surgery was so successful, here's what would happen.

I'd go into his office feeling very proud of my new abilities and say to him something like, "This is great! I'm normal!" He couldn't wait to catch me on this one, "Wait a minute! Don't get carried away, Leanne! I said that we may be able to make you seizure free. Now I never said that we could make you normal!" He'd kind of chuckle as he said this, and then end with a big laugh. You knew you were on his good list when you were not "normal." He'd often make comments like, "Who wants to be normal?" and "Now cheer up, kiddo!" and "Are you going to be okay? You have to tell me you are going to be okay before you leave!"

I sure didn't like people making decisions with my life, but there was some kind of reassurance that I got after seeing Dr. Leroy. He has this, "everything is going to be fine" attitude. I suppose with his job if he didn't have that attitude, he wouldn't be too successful. He sees some really messed up people. And I mean no disrespect in saying that. I'm just pointing out that he often gets the patients in difficult situations and the patients that other doctors may be "too busy" for.

I think that physicians, the good ones, and their patients, who try their hardest to overcome illness, have a lot in common. I never saw this until after surgery. I always felt like my doctors were these really important people who had to make really important decisions, and patients, including myself, were in this other category of beings.

I don't feel that way any more. First off, doctors may be patients, too, and they also have to go to other physicians when they have problems. Second, most good physicians are good because they work at being good. It's not like they acquire this status with a medical degree and that's all it takes. It's very demanding work, and if they don't keep up with the changing world of medicine, that degree isn't going to do them much good.

They have to go to continuing educational classes for credits that are requirements for maintaining their status, and they often have to be on call on their days off. The similarity that I have noticed with physicians and their patients is that both have to work awfully hard in order to do well. Patients struggle with a medical problem, and physicians struggle with the changing world of medicine and the demands placed on them by the medical board, the hospital, and the health insurance companies.

Physicians are married to their work and patients are stuck in a bad relationship with a disease, illness, or disability. Neither gets much time off. Both the physician and the patient must have a sense of humor about life in order to get through the struggles they face. Laughing about life is a way of releasing the stress, and both must be able to do it appropriately if they want to succeed. Laughing at the wrong times can cost the doctor his/her job and cause the patient more stress.

The relationship between physician and patient is very symbiotic. We need each other, plain and simple, no matter how much one of us doesn't like it. We have to learn to get along, and we have to learn to work together.

Where is this going? I'll tell you. Never in my adult life did I feel like I had to depend on people in ways that I did not choose. Having epilepsy forced me into situations where I was absolutely powerless, and it was one of the worse feelings in the world. It's like you are young and healthy, but you are still vulnerable. It's like being old but in a young body. Your short-term memory doesn't always work too well, the medication keeps you lethargic, you aren't supposed to drive, people may try to take advantage of you, and you will be confused for a couple of days after grand mal seizures. It's funny, but maybe one good thing about having lived with epilepsy is that now I'm not afraid to get old.

Triumph

It's about time, it's about life
It's the pain that you hide.
It's the anger, the frustration,
that eats you up inside.

It's the love for the hunger,
and the feelings you deny.
It's the drive to conquer.
It's the race to win,
too many to fight,
too few to give in.

It's the freedom, it's the spirit
and learning how to play.
It's the beginning of the game
and the end of the day.
It's passion that gives its heart away.

It's about triumph over matter
the love for something you crave.
It's survival, the need to win,
it's humiliation and fitting in.
It's anger and pain
and frustration, once again.
No longer needing to play,
You win!

12/21/98

Σ

34. Freedom

What is Freedom?

Freedom is a big word for people with epilepsy. I'm hoping that some of the people who bought this book who do not have seizures will pay particular attention to this chapter. If you are the person with epilepsy, please let someone in your life read this. I think they will have a better understanding of what freedom is to us.

So What Is Freedom?

Freedom...is the opportunity to walk down a public street without intense fear that within the next half-hour you may be in an emergency room somewhere.

Freedom...is the ability to lay down in your bed at night, knowing that...when you wake up in the morning you will remember the people closest to you, you will not have blood on your pillows and sheets from biting your tongue during an attack, your muscles will not be sore from convulsing, you will not stutter during the day trying to find the words you need to express your thoughts, you will not have blackouts, and you will not have to worry that you will be so brain-damaged that you may not want to live any more.

Freedom...is forgetting something and knowing that it will come back to you later.

Freedom...is sitting in a room full of strangers and not having to worry about whom to trust to take care of you when your brain decides to check out.

Freedom...is going through an entire day without having to worry about when and where to take your medication.

Freedom...is not having to worry that you forgot to take your medication or that you left it at home when you walked out of the house this morning.

Freedom...is knowing that you can travel anywhere you want to and not have to keep your neurologist's emergency number attached to your person twenty-four hours a day.

Freedom...is knowing that you can get into your car and drive it anywhere you want to, whenever you want to, and for as long as you want to.

Freedom...is knowing that you don't have a psychological problem that is causing your body to convulse uncontrollably in the night.

Freedom...is knowing that you can get a job anywhere and not have to worry that you will be fired because your brain does not work properly.

And finally,

Freedom...is letting go of the past and going on with your life.

Σ

35. *Four Years Seizure Free*

Two years ago, I bought a nice, big house with a swimming pool. That was my goal twelve years ago when I started doing hair shows. I thought I was going to travel around the world making money by teaching people my wonderful knowledge (that of course only I possessed) about how to take care of their hair. I didn't know that epilepsy would force me out of self-employment, and I also didn't know that I'd discover the superficial world that I was living in. I guess it's a good thing that I started having seizures.

Now I have two books published, and I'm working on a third one. I've met some very good people with very good hearts. I've also lived in a place that most won't even come close to. Old age may be similar, but not the same.

It's kind of weird how things turn out, isn't it? You think you are going down one road to get what you want, and a different road ends up taking you there. Maybe fate has something to do with it. Maybe we are destined to go somewhere, but how we get there may have nothing to do with our goals or our beliefs at the time. Maybe we are destined to end up in a certain place by nature of our very beings. And maybe this is just the beginning of my life.

Perhaps, epilepsy, as big as it seemed at the time is only the beginning. Maybe I will be in a completely different world in several more years from now. What matters the most is that I make a difference because of what happened in my life. What matters is that I was able to create something that perhaps gave someone else comfort on their road to self-acceptance and to recovery. I'd like to do more with my life, and I'd like to remember that whatever happens from here, I'm no longer alone. You've traveled this journey with me now, and it's over.

We can say goodbye to the past and welcome the new opportunities without regret. I can look back on my life and feel very fortunate. I can feel grateful for the people who were there for me and who felt special in my life.

The dynamics of my relationships have changed, with my friends, with my family, with my environment, and with the world. I can understand that this is a natural growing process for most people. I also understand that when a person suffers a traumatic life style change, the maturing process is temporarily put on hold. When we get well, it's like we age overnight. We have to change a lot if we want to fit in, and then we have to re-learn how to handle people and how to handle situations. The problem with this is that within a few short years, we feel very old. We go through a lot in a short period of time, and we feel old afterwards. Unfortunately, there's not much we can do about that part. We just have to find a new way to get meaning from our lives, so we don't continue feeling old.

I did go back to doing hair for a short while, and I enjoyed my clients and our conversations, just like before, but somehow, it wasn't the same. Somewhere along the way, my perception of the business and my perception of myself had changed. That was the good news and the bad news, both, because that also meant I could no longer get the same gratification that I did before, from doing the same things. The meaning out of doing hair and being in the salon was lost when I got well. I didn't want to lose that! My life had changed, and the significance of my previous activities had to change with it.

I found out some other things about this adventure that I am only just now becoming aware of. Kay had some feelings of her own that she wanted to share with me. We decided to put her feelings in the book for those readers who have friends or family with epilepsy. Perhaps her thoughts will validate some of your feelings and help you, as well!

Septemb

Hey Lee-Lee!

    Well, you are probably wondering "why the fax?" Well, it's sort of like this: I just finished reading your entire book this very minute, and all I could think was, "WOW!!!!!" And I mean all of it, too (not just the parts that I am in--although those are my personal favorites).

    I loved your willingness to share about the really tough times as well as the awkward funny anecdotes that had me laughing out loud to myself! I am so so so glad that you wrote this book even if for your own therapy, and that you printed it so that other people could benefit from your experience and from your insight as well. I know, because I am one of those people who benefited from it!

    Believe it or not, as I was traveling through your journey with having epilepsy, dealing with the epilepsy, and learning to live with and without the epilepsy, my mind couldn't help but wander off and remember a time when I was going through my own journey. As you, yourself, alluded to in your poem, "Ode To A Bad Relationship." And in a very comical way, but yet real way, you took me emotionally through my journey with having a husband, dealing with that husband, and learning to live with and without that husband, without taking away from the obvious differences involved between having a husband versus having a presumably incurable, life-threatening disease.

    If you could take me to a place emotionally that would draw up all sorts of memories and images just from being married, can you imagine how many freaked- out that would have made me feel had our roles been reversed!!! I didn't need to add drama to the already tense situation.

I guess I had blocked out all of those thoughts previously because I was more afraid of what would happen to you if you kept on with a lifetime of seizures and medication. I was more afraid of losing my sister as I knew you, with a fully functioning alert and non-damaged brain! The thought of losing you to this affliction had been such an ongoing and great fear that all I could focus on was how you were going to get better!

Anyway, as I was saying, the moment you took the "goofy juice" is when I remember distinctly what was going through my head--all fear! I'll tell you now, but obviously it's a good thing I didn't mention these things at that time. What if the knife slipped (and I mean no disrespect to the brilliant and competent Dr. Bruce)? What if they took the wrong piece out of your brain? Or what if they took too much of your brain out? Or what if they took out the part that had your personality on it? Would you be the same person? Or worse yet, what if they accidentally erased a part of your long-term memory? Would you remember all of the funny things we used to laugh about, like "Buenos" and "Spatula'" and "Mi familia y mi go to Fort Myers" and especially, "5 weeks!!!"

What if somehow the competent surgeon wiped out all of this "stuff" with one deft stroke of the scalpel? And where would that leave me with my sister? Would you even remember me? And even then I felt a little guilty for thinking about all of that since it was you who was getting a "new lease on life." And how could I be thinking of myself at a time like this and how all of that would affect me? So, now you know what I was really thinking.

I haven't thought about that for a long time. Obviously your book brought back a lot of memories for me as well. So, while you were drinking your "juice," when all of that hit me, that is exactly when I quickly grabbed the video camera and started filming you and joking about how I was going to blackmail you with it later. I was hoping that as soon as we started laughing again, I would be able to hold it together, at least until they knocked you out. And I suppose it worked for the most part.

But the next thing that happened took me over the edge after all. I might have told you this already, but when you first came out of surgery we were allowed to go in and see you in the ICU, one at a time. Well, you were all hooked up to the machinery paraphernalia, with electrodes and wires sticking out all over you, not to mention the bizarre looking incision mark all jagged across your lobe! I also didn't know at the time that Dr. Bruce "meant" to do that. From where I was standing it just looked like your ingenious surgeon had a very shaky cutting hand (so I could only imagine what else that might mean).

Anyway, I was standing there looking at you, waiting for you to move or speak or do anything, and suddenly you opened your eyes, looked kind of at me, and then shut them again. And just as you this, some alarm went off on your equipment and started wailing out this obnoxiously loud warning siren. You didn't move or twitch or do anything. The nurse pushed me back out of the way, and a team of nurses started checking all of your vitals instantly. And that's when I lost it!

I had to run to the bathroom because I was so

scared of what might happen, and I couldn't stop crying for a long time! I even got so nauseated that I thought I was going to throw up. So much for holding it together, huh?

Well, I'm glad I can tell you about it now. Shortly thereafter they discovered what the alarm was all about. Apparently when you woke up, you moved ever so slightly and dislodged one of the many electrodes attached to you, so it wasn't an emergency after all. Thank God!

So, in concluding, let me just say that I am soooooooooo glad that whole ordeal is in the past. And fortunately time helps you forget the things you don't want to think about. But I'm so glad that I got a chance to relive that whole ordeal again (with your book) because it reminded me of how much I have to be grateful for now. For one, I still have the best sister in my life, and two, you actually have a life now!

It scared me all over again just reading the book, and I wanted to make sure you know how lucky I feel to still have you here with me , struggling through our lives, and wading through the "what do I want to be when I grow up" waters together. And I thank God for that!

I love you, Lee Lee. Thanks for writing such a great book!

Love,
Goo

Before we go, I'd like to comment on what Kay said about my incision. Dr. Bruce makes the incision with a jagged line so that the scar will be less obvious when it heals. The scar will remain pink for about four to six months and then gradually turn white. If I want to see my scar I can, but the nice part is that I don't have to.

I'd also like to point out that I did not have to get my head shaved. This technique is supposed to help prevent the onset of infection after surgery. When the head is shaved, it's easier for the surgeon, but also increases the chance of infection for the patient. I don't know if the chance of infection is of a significant risk, but the patients usually like to keep their hair. You will need to ask the surgeon what his/her preference is for doing your type of surgery, as they all have their own techniques they like to use and their own reasons for using them.

But I will tell you that there is one minor drawback to not having your head shaved. By the time you leave the hospital, you will probably look pretty normal. I looked no different when I left the hospital than I did when I entered it. I had a jagged mark across my temporal lobe, but it wasn't too noticeable. I was walking slowly and cautiously, and probably acting a little weird, but I looked normal.

There's a psychological aspect to healing as we discussed earlier. There is also a psychological effect that creates confusion in our minds when we look good, but feel so bad. It's hard to accept feeling bad, when you look like you should be recovered already. I guess it just goes back to being patient and remembering to remind yourself that you've had a part of your brain removed, and you will need some time to heal.

I'd say that being patient is maybe fifty percent of the healing process, but believing in yourself is the other fifty percent. If you believe that you can make it, you will. We all agree that we need good surgeons. I'm only giving you advice based on what you can do and what responsibility you can take, assuming your surgeon has given you the best possible chance for a better life. The point is that no matter how good our surgeons are, we are still ultimately responsible for making the adjustments and for making something of ourselves. And this applies to everyone!

The problem is that most of us think in terms of limitations in life, regardless of whether we have an illness or we've had surgery or we've had some other traumatic experience. And you absolutely have to believe that you can succeed or at least be able to convince everyone else around you that you can, if you really want to. The minute you start placing limitations on life or on yourself, you stop looking for creative outlets for accomplishing your goals. In life there will always be challenges to face, and if you limit the outcome of your choices, you may miss the way out! That's the advice I'd like to give anyone who would like to change something in their lives.

It's not about who is the richest, or the strongest, or the smartest, or who is given the most. It's about who can face obstacles and succeed against all odds. It's about how you handle life's circumstances and what you do with what you have. It's about doing the best you can, when you want nothing more than to quit! It's about how you handle people and how you handle yourself! It's about making a difference and feeling good about what you've done.

I wrote *Seizure Free,* trying to solve some of my own problems I suppose. However, after I published it, I began to slowly feel better. I wasn't sure how people would react to my book, and I was terrified of the rejection I would get as a result of publishing such personal and questionable material. After all, this wasn't just a book, this was my life--the most private and precious part of my youth that I shared with only a hand full of people. But I decided to take the risk because I felt like it was all that I had to offer the world. I knew how to survive, and I did it really well! Now it was my time to give something back!

Although I did get some rejection and weird reactions when I talked about my book, for the most part, everyone was very supportive and very helpful. My goal was to make a difference, and I believe that I am now accomplishing that. This is the second edition of *Seizure Free,* and I'm glad to say that we have just about sold out of the first edition. I know that I shouldn't brag but it's kind of exciting to see a project that you have put all of your feelings into come alive.

When I had epilepsy, most of my money went to medical bills. I learned how to invest , how to be frugal, and how to live on a budget. My only luxury investment was a new pair of running shoes every year. I know exactly what it feels like not to be able to have what you want, but unfortunately, you can't take out a loan to get your life back. You just have to work very hard and be very lucky! The second one I can't help you with, sorry!

Thanks to my parents I learned some very good lessons early in life. If you don't have the money, don't buy it! Don't pay for things on credit if you can't pay off the bill when it comes in, and always invest a little of what you have no matter how much you make. It's funny how these things come back to you as you get older. Follow a few simple rules, have a little self-discipline, and you will be able to do anything financially!

So I tried to take care of my money, and I didn't talk much about the seizures when I was having them. I didn't even tell too many people that I had epilepsy. It was like the big "E" word was not in my vocabulary.

Four years postop (after surgery), and I can now say the word epilepsy without getting nauseated. It has taken me a very long time to get to this point, however!

I do still have issues, but probably not too unlike anyone else in this world. And I can say that I have learned a few things in life along the way. It's important to understand that everyone has issues. No matter how wealthy, how fit, how strong, how intelligent, how successful, or how positive we are, we all have issues!

I suppose we just have to look at life and try to decide what we can live with and what we can't live with. We try to change the things we can't live with, we try to accept the things that we decide to live with, and we try to work for the things that we want to live with.

Maybe life isn't as complicated as it seems, but somehow when our feelings get involved, everything gets all messed up. I had a lot of feelings about getting epilepsy, and I also had a lot of challenges to face with it. I don't know that I did everything the right way or even if there is a right way, but I do know that I have something to offer.

I know that since surgery, I've learn something new everyday and my perspective has been growing constantly, as well. I know that I can tell you how I did it, and what I've learned along the way. I can give you advice and suggestions that might make it easier for you so that you don't have to go through the pain and mental anguish alone. I'm right here with you!

I also learned that writing can be very rewarding and very therapeutic for the writer, but unless it helps someone else in some kind of way, what's the point? Personally, I think that writing is a very selfish process. It involves zero communication and no interaction with anyone else. Mostly it's a way to make the writer feel better about something, or to boost the writer's ego.

Now before I convince you that I am just a selfish person after nothing more than an ego boost for seeing my thoughts in print, I will tell you something else. Putting my feelings and my personal life on paper for the world to critique has not been easy. Yes, I have received favorable comments on *Seizure Free*, but the risk I took was huge. Not even my parents knew about a lot of this stuff, and I had to warn them before the book came out. Sharing this information has been one of the hardest things I've ever done, but knowing that my experience and my thoughts have made a difference for someone else is the gratification that has made this whole process worthwhile.

I want to thank you for taking the time to read my book and for being a part of my life. I hope you got something positive out of my story that you will be able to take with you on your own journey. I wish you the very best in obtaining whatever it is you are looking for. And don't forget...Have Fun!

ORDER FORM

For extra copies of *SEIZURE FREE, 2nd Edition, Revised*
please send check or money order to:
> ENGLISH PRESS PUBLICATIONS
> PO Box 742945
> Dallas, TX 75374

For Credit Card Orders, Please call 1-888-357-1135
or visit us on the web at **www.EnglishPress.com**

_____ SEIZURE FREE @ $12.95 each $_____

_____ Please send book/s to the person/s below

OR

_____ Please send book/s as a gift to person/s below

(gift wrap +card "compliments

of [your name]" add $ 2.95) $_____

(Texas residents add 8.25% sales tax to order) $_____

shipping: $1.95 book rate (7-10 days)

$2.95 first class (3-5 days)

$3.95 priority (2-3 days)

+ flat rate of $.95 for each additional book $_____

Total enclosed: $_____

Name: _____

Address: _____

City:_____ State:_____ Zip:_____

We want your thoughts!
Please leave your comments at
englishpress@prodigy.net
and your review will be posted to our web page.

SEIZURE FREE

*From Epilepsy to Brain Surgery,
I Survived, and You Can, Too!*

LEANNE CHILTON

ΣNGLISH PRESS PUBLICATIONS

SEIZURE FREE

Published by: English Press Publications
                PO Box 742945
                Dallas, TX 75374
                214-349-4441 (phone)
                214-349-4241 (fax)
                888-357-1135 (voice)

                www.EnglishPress.com
                englishpress@prodigy.net

Copyright: 1998 by Leanne Chilton
             2000, Second Edition, Revised
             by Leanne Chilton

ISBN 0-9663819-0-4
Library of Congress Catalog Card Number: 99-90708

Printed by: Malloy Lithographing, Inc.